HOW CAN I MAKE IT BETTER?

A guide to pain management
for day surgery nurses

HOW CAN I MAKE IT BETTER?
A guide to pain management for day surgery nurses

Anne Marie Coll

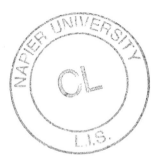

Fivepin

APS Publishing
Fivepin Limited, 91 Crane Street, Salisbury, Wiltshire, SP1 2PU
www.apspublishing.co.uk

British Library Cataloguing in Publication Data
A catalogue record for this book is available from the British
Library

© Fivepin Limited 2006
ISBN 1 9038773 7 7

Printed in the United Kingdom by Lightning Source UK Limited,
Milton Keynes

Contents

Contents

Acknowledgements

This book would not have been possible without the unfailing support, invaluable advice and friendship of Dr Jamal Ameen and Mrs Roswyn Hakesley-Brown in the designing and writing of the book and Mr Lyn Harris the cartoonist. A special word of thanks also to Dr Ian Jackson for the expert advice.

List of Illustrations and Tables

List of Cartoons

List of Figures

List of Tables

Foreword

By writing this guide, Dr Coll has already made a significant contribution to making pain better after day surgery and is to be congratulated. Day surgery nurses should find this important text invaluable in informing their day-to-day professional practice. Whilst day surgery makes good economic and technical sense, we have to ensure that it makes 'quality of patient care' sense too, in every aspect. Innovative medical approaches to surgical interventions will be pointless if the patient experience is compromised by the utter misery of intractable pain in the domestic situation on discharge from hospital.

Witnessing the severe and sometimes excruciating discomfort of loved ones should not be a burden of care for the significant others of day surgery patients. The publication of this text should make that kind of distressing scenario a thing of the past. Managing pain is a complex activity and requires high level skills to get it right. It is particularly important for day surgery patients who do not continue their care in the secure confines of the hospital ward. The management of pain after discharge must not be left to chance and/or the good offices of primary care staff.

This important text has the potential to liberate the skills of the multidisciplinary team as well as to operationalise the true spirit of effective patient/family partnerships. Hearing what patients say and acting on that communication is an essential component of the patient/professional relationship. Having the knowledge and confidence to plan for the enduring comfort of the patient carries with it the satisfaction of a job well done.

I have vivid recollections of agonising pain following major surgery to my neck and asking a nurse for aspirin because of my lifelong fear of needles! No one knew that and never asked, or carried out an assessment. Perhaps some national guidelines for pain relief are long overdue and this book will set the ball rolling. In my view, given my painful experiences, this can't happen soon enough. It is with a sense of great relief that I look forward to seeing this text on every nursing library bookshelf.

Effective pain management is every day surgery nurses' business. This book, thankfully, will help to make it so!

Mrs Roswyn Hakesley-Brown
Ex-President, Royal College of Nursing

Introduction

'I thought I was going to die, I felt dreadful and I am thinking they're kicking me out now, and I felt as though I was being kicked out, like the place was closing, the cleaners were going around and I thought, "Oh, I shouldn't be here."'

(Patient A)

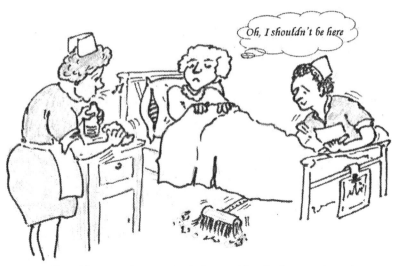

"...I felt as though I was being kicked out, like the place was closing"

Cartoon 0.1: Feeling under pressure to leave

Does this sound familiar? For this woman who had undergone laparoscopic sterilisation, the day surgery experience proved to be very distressing and painful. This is not

uncommon. Evidence suggests that severe pain for this procedure can persist until the seventh postoperative day (Agboola
et al, 1999; Coll, 2001). As a day surgery nurse myself, I was
only too aware of the problem of severe pain experience after
day surgery. Possibly, due to the short time spent in hospital,
patients equated what they considered to be a minor procedure (because they were in and out on the same day) with
minor symptoms. They were therefore not prepared for the
severe pain they went on to experience which, more often
than not, was likely to take place at home afterwards.

During my years of practice, I was aware that patients were
being discharged home whilst still experiencing significantly
high levels of pain. As I recall, there were several contributory
factors:

- Patents were not well informed at their pre-operative
  assessment for the likelihood of pain experience (we all
  know that thorough pre-operative preparation results in
  less anxiety and post-operative pain (Barthelsson *et al*,
  2003a;b; Dewar *et al*, 2003; Moore *et al*, 2002; Skilton,
  2003);

- The unit closed every evening, thus, if the patient was not
  able to return home, the likelihood of finding a bed within
  the main hospital was difficult, particularly on a Friday
  afternoon or if the hospital was on emergency intake;

- The patient wanted to return home to the comfort of their
  own bed or to care for their dependents.

My main concern related to how these patients coped at home
during their post-operative period. Unless there was an emergency re-admission (which was rare), or the district nurse
contacted us with a problem (if the patient had needed to be
referred), there was no routine follow-up. Consequently, we
never heard from these patients again. This was an important
aspect of continuity of care that was omitted. The question I
often asked myself was 'Do patients suffer unnecessarily at

home after their discharge?' This proved to be the main incentive for the research I subsequently carried out.

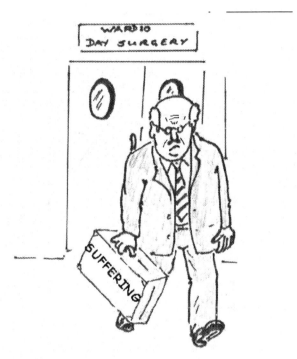

..do patients suffer unnecessarily at home after their discharge?

Cartoon 0.2: Unnecessary suffering after day surgery

This book, therefore, has taken an evidence-based approach combining both my own research findings and those of others specifically related to patients' experience of pain after day surgery. Evidence is presented which suggests that nurses could be better assessors and managers of pain and recommendations are made for how these skills can be improved. It is an essential guide for all day surgery nurses and it is not intended as an academic text book but a more practical cartoon-based approach with the aim of ultimately improving the day surgery experience for the patient.

How this book is organised

Chapter 1 presents a definition of day surgery and briefly looks at its development within the UK. The problem of pain experience is introduced as well as its impact on the patient, their family members and the primary healthcare team. Chapter 2 deals with the pain phenomenon incorporating a holistic approach with physiological, psychological and social explanations. The multidimensionality of pain is then described and a review of pain assessment tools used in measuring the different components of it is presented. Chapter 3 offers a literature review of the evidence on pain experience after day surgery in which three salient issues are highlighted:

- Severe pain experience after day surgery occurs despite advancements in analgesia and anaesthesia;

- Many pain assessment tools have been established to measure different components of pain, which has led to a diversity in reported levels of pain afterwards; and

- There are disparities in reported levels of pain within different surgical specialities and in relation to specific operative procedures; thus 'acceptable' levels of pain following day surgery have not been established.

Chapter 4 tackles the issue of the responsibility of the qualified nurse and his/her role in the management of pain after day surgery and looks more closely at the evidence. It is suggested that nurses could do more to alleviate their patients' pain but there are barriers which both the nurse and the patient bring to their encounter with each other. Chapter 5 adopts a practical approach and makes recommendations for how nurses can improve their pain assessment and management skills from preparing the patient pre-operatively for a realistic expectation of the procedure and expected pain levels, through to their follow-up management after discharge. The final chapter briefly considers the future of day surgery, including the increasing trend of expansion to more complex surgery and other policy imperatives. The success of the day surgery process can only be ensured if post-operative pain, even for the most common procedures, is effectively managed first.

How to use this book

At the beginning of each chapter, a list of learning outcomes is presented. These are otherwise known as learning goals and you should be able to achieve them by the end of each chapter. I have also included some further reading to help you consolidate your learning. Each chapter represents an independent

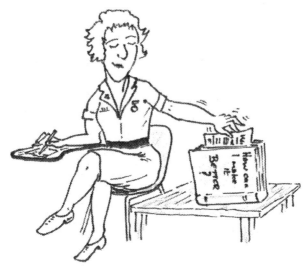

...you can 'dip' into the book at leisure

Cartoon 0.3: Dipping into the book at leisure

section of the book thus you can 'dip' into the book at leisure depending on the area of interest, so you are not obliged to start at the beginning.

Do patients still experience pain after day surgery?

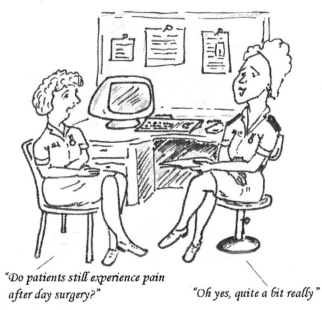

"*Do patients still experience pain after day surgery?*"

"*Oh yes, quite a bit really*"

Cartoon 1.1: Do patients experience pain after day surgery?

Learning outcomes

At the end of this chapter, the nurse will be aware of:

- The definitions of 'day surgery';
- The development of day surgery in relation to the technological advancements in anaesthesia and analgesia; and

- The influence of post-operative pain on day surgery patients, their family members and the primary healthcare team.

Definitions and the development of day surgery

Looking back to the development of day surgery, it seems that the concept of hospital surgery without a subsequent inpatient stay only occurred during the 1970s, although we do know that as early as 1909, James Nicholl, a paediatric surgeon, routinely carried out surgical procedures on children on an outpatient basis. Since then, there has been a dramatic expansion in the use of day surgery (Wetchler, 1997) with the development of under 24 hours day surgery. Indeed, the National Health Service (NHS) Plan (Dept of Health, 2000) has a stated target of achieving three quarters of all elective operations to be performed as day surgery by 2010 with many day surgery units already achieving this (Department of Health, 2002). By comparison, day surgery in the US constituted 60–70 per cent of all surgery in the 1990s and continues to increase (Chung et al, 1997; Marley and Swanson, 2001).

The Royal College of Surgeons in England defines day surgery as 'a patient who is admitted for investigation or an operation on a planned non resident basis and who none-the-less requires facilities for recovery' (McHugh and Thoms, 2002). Jackson and McWhinnie (2002) define it in two ways. The first definition is that of: 'any patient who manages to meet discharge criteria within 12 hours of the end of the operation' and the second, there is under 24 hour or Ambulatory Surgery which is defined to incorporate an overnight stay and includes: 'any patient treated in a designated facility by designated staff and discharged within 24 hours of admission'. This development has meant that more complex surgery due to technological developments in surgery and anaesthesia can now be performed. For example, laparoscopic cholecystectomy and vaginal hysterectomy can be carried out, as well as the more common procedures, such as cataract and hernia surgery, on those patients once considered unsuitable as they no longer need to have a carer to look after them overnight. Furthermore, given the increase in hospital-acquired infections (especially Methicillin-resistant *Staphylococcus aureus*, MRSA), day surgery is becoming increasingly more attractive, not only to the commissioners, but also to the patient.

However, the concept of under 24 hour surgery has only become more popular in recent years. During the mid 1990s, for me and many other day surgery nurses, day surgery meant 'half day' surgery during which a morning and afternoon operative list was performed. At that time, with the exception of hernia and varicose vein patients, most morning patients were expected to be discharged before the arrival of the afternoon patients so that the necessary beds were available.

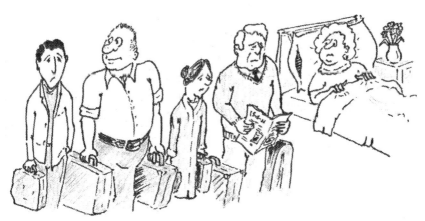

...most patients were expected to be discharged before the arrival of the afternoon patients

Cartoon 1.2: Half day surgery

Of course, the success of the day surgery process is dependent on patients who have been appropriately selected. Most day surgery units now have their own pre-operative assessment template, although their criteria are based on those devised by the American Society of Anesthesiologists (ASA, 1963) and include selection factors of physical status, class, age, weight and general good health. We know that, to all intents and purposes, the day surgery population is healthy except for the elective surgical intervention they need, such as the request to be sterilised or to have an inguinal hernia repair. They will include both male and female, a range of ages (from six months to 90 years) and different socioeconomic status and educational ability. The day surgery process cannot be successful if patients undergoing a general anaesthetic have a pre-existing condition such as diabetes, a chronic chest problem or have experienced a recent angina attack or epileptic episode, as they are expected to return home the same day and resume their activities soon afterwards.

The main rationale for the development of day surgery, therefore, clearly rests on three main contributory factors:

- Technological advancements in medical practice;

- A current practice in favour of earlier ambulation, shorter hospitalisation; and

- More cost effectiveness than in-patient surgery.

Pain experience after day surgery

Within anaesthetics, technological advancements have developed shorter acting anaesthetics (Wigens, 1997), stronger orally administered analgesia (Chung et al, 1997) and minimal access surgery to reduce the traumatic insult to the patient (Banta, 1993; Cushieri, 1999). It could be assumed, therefore, that, as a result of these advancements, pain after day surgery would be minimal. Yet, surprisingly, this is not the case. In the literature doubts have been voiced about the effects that this rapid growth has had on the pain experienced by patients having day surgery (Boey, 1995; Marshall and Chung, 1997). The experience of pain and the effects due to the administration of analgesia are the most common problems before discharge and during the first 24 hours afterwards (McMenemin, 1999; Mitchell, 2004). It has also been shown that patients continue to experience pain at a severe level on the third post-operative day (Coll, 2001), the fourth (McHugh and Thoms, 2002) and as late as the seventh post-operative day (Agboola, 1999; Beauregard et al, 1998). The most common problems associated with severe pain experience that have been identified so far have included:

• Delayed discharge (Chung, 1995; Joshi, 1994);

• Unplanned contact with the GP (Ghosh and Sallam, 1994; Kong et al, 1997); and

• Unanticipated re-admission (Fortier et al, 1996; Gold et al, 1989).

As Kiley (2004: 7) has described it:

'If we think ourselves as more sophisticated in therapies of pain today, the alarming statistics may raise a few eyebrows Pain is still the single biggest health concern; it is the single most common complaint brought to our doctors and our medicine cabinets are choked full of remedies to quiet the aches and pains of our ailing modern bodies.'

Clearly the effects of severe pain experience will not only impact on the patient, but also on their families, as well as the primary healthcare team. The increased rate of day surgery is no doubt achieved at some cost to the patient's family. For example, as the comment from the cartoon at the beginning of this chapter suggests, it has been shown that, for laparoscopic sterilisation patients, they:

• Were unprepared for their day surgery experience (Rudkin et al, 1993);

- Had unrealistic expectations about how much recovery time was needed after discharge (Thomas and Hare, 1987);
- Were not prepared for the severity of pain experienced (Cooper *et al*, 1995); and
- Had needed physical and emotional support afterwards (Cooper *et al*, 1995).

Ultimately, the patient's family will be faced with the physical and psychological costs of this continuing care.

With respect to the increased burden on the primary healthcare team, it appears that post-operative problems of pain (Jackson *et al*, 1993; Kong *et al*, 1997) and wound infection (Bailey *et al*, 1992; Willis *et al*, 1997) are cited as the main reasons for GP contact after discharge from day surgery. Surprisingly, few studies have considered the views of district nurses with regard to the impact on their workload (Kelly, 1994). However, with the expansion of more ambitious surgery in the future, this will inevitably result in a greater demand on the primary healthcare team (Kelly *et al*, 1998; Lewis and Bryson, 1998).

So what can we, as nurses, do to improve the situation? As healthcare professionals, we have a duty of care to our patients and as the patient's advocate (NMC, 2002), our fundamental responsibility is in the effective assessment and management of pain, so that the patient has what could be described as an acceptable level of pain. Before we can attempt to assess and holistically manage this concept, it is important to first understand what pain is. What is clear is that its subjectiveness of character, and the complexity of feelings it evokes, make its reliable measurement by healthcare professionals a challenge in its successful management.

Summary

Day surgery has been defined as the performance of an elective procedure in which the patient returns home on the same day or within 24 hours of the procedure. The technological advancements in both anaesthesia and analgesia are major factors which have contributed to the development of day surgery and the complexity of different and exciting surgical techniques such as laparoscopic cholecystectomy. By 2010 it is anticipated that three quarters of all elective surgery will be performed as day surgery.

Uncontrolled pain is the major symptom experienced by patients, particularly after being discharged home. Thus, it is not clear to what extent day surgery patients suffer unnecessarily, although it can be argued that, to a larger extent, family members and, to a lesser extent, the primary healthcare team will carry this burden.

In Chapter 2, we examine the pain phenomenon and define it by incorporating a holistic approach based on physiological, psychological and social explanations. Pain as a multidimensional concept is introduced and a brief review of the most widely used pain assessment tools in accommodating its multidimensions is described.

Further reading

Department of Health (2002) *Day Surgery: Operational Guide: Waiting, Booking and Choice.* DoH, London

Hodge D (1998) *Day Surgery: A Nursing Approach.* Blackwell, Oxford

Penn S, Davenport TH, Carrington S *et al* (1996) *Principles of Day Surgery Nursing.* Blackwell, Oxford

2

What is pain anyway?

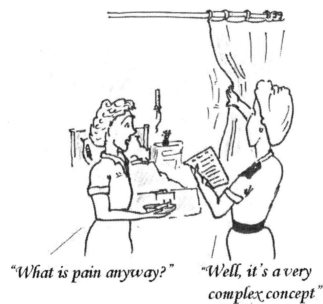

"What is pain anyway?" *"Well, it's a very complex concept"*

Cartoon 2.1: What is pain anyway?

Learning outcomes

At the end of this chapter, the nurse will be able to:

- Provide a definition of pain;
- Understand the pain phenomenon in the context of a total experience using a bio-psychosocial approach incorporating the physiological, sensory, affective, cognitive, behavioural and socio-cultural dimensions;
- Understand the importance of pain assessment; and

- Review the use of pain assessment tools in his/her own clinical area of day surgery practice.

Introduction

So what does the word 'pain' mean to you? We know that pain is a universal phenomenon which is experienced by everyone irrespective of age, socioeconomic status, gender and country of birth. Pain could be described as a nebulous complex concept having several definitions and dimensions. I am sure that you have heard pain described as a 'multidimensional' concept. This is because pain is a total experience affecting the individual physically, psychologically and socially. So, it is clear that the experience is not simply the intensity of the painful stimulus you feel, but how you perceive it, and factors such as previous experiences of pain, socialisation and personality will influence personal pain thresholds. McCaffery and Beebe's (1989: 7) famous phrase 'Pain is whatever the experiencing person says it is and exists whenever they say it does' pays tribute to the uniqueness and individuality of this perception. An excellent analogy of pain is used by Daudet (2002; cited by Fitzgerald, 2004) when he describes how the nature of pain varies 'like a singer's voice according to the acoustics of the hall'. So pain has a personal meaning for every one of us.

Definitions of pain

For many years, and certainly up to the 1960s, pain was defined as an objective sensory response (Loeser, 2004). However, further research, including work by Melzack and Casey (1968), established that pain was no longer a sensory response to a stimulus only, but that there would also be a reactive element to it which would also involve an emotional response. This definition was later adopted by the

International Association for the Study of Pain (1994) and forms the basis of its definition.

The contemporary definition of pain is one where the sensory and emotional response is experienced by the person in a unique and individual way so that pain becomes a personal and subjective experience. Therefore, the uniqueness of this experience is not only shaped by the person's physical functioning, but also by their:

- Emotions;
- Work;
- Family;
- Behaviour; and
- Socio-cultural background (see *Figure 2.1*).

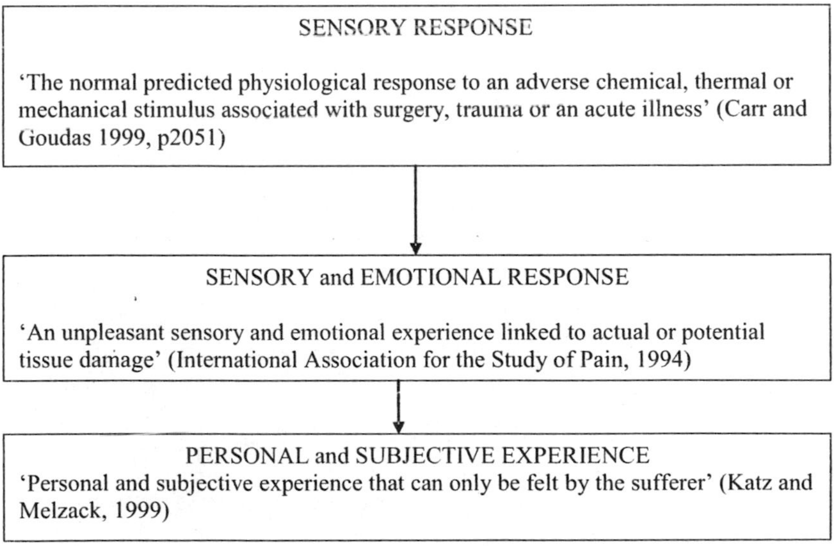

SENSORY RESPONSE

'The normal predicted physiological response to an adverse chemical, thermal or mechanical stimulus associated with surgery, trauma or an acute illness' (Carr and Goudas 1999, p2051)

↓

SENSORY and EMOTIONAL RESPONSE

'An unpleasant sensory and emotional experience linked to actual or potential tissue damage' (International Association for the Study of Pain, 1994)

↓

PERSONAL and SUBJECTIVE EXPERIENCE
'Personal and subjective experience that can only be felt by the sufferer' (Katz and Melzack, 1999)

Figure 2.1: Definitions of pain

Thus, everyone will feel pain differently because the individual's perception of it will tap into their unique emotional, social, familial and occupational, as well as their physical, functioning.

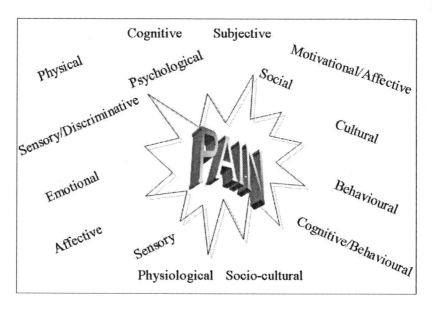

Cartoon 2.2: Dimensions of pain

The range of terminologies listed above demonstrates how differently a variety of researchers have interpreted pain. As you can see, this diversity in the definitions and dimensions of the pain, has led to the use of a variety of pain measurement tools to capture the experience. These different measurement tools have led, in turn, to different assessments and measures of pain and hence difficulty in reliably assessing and managing it. For example, do you know what the average level of pain experience is after laparoscopic sterilisation and for how long it is likely to continue? The problem of reporting pain will be discussed further in the next chapter.

Physiological dimension

It is now useful to consider pain within the context of its different dimensions by first considering its physical, neurologic and biochemical aspects. The physiological inflammatory response of the body to pain is usually the result of trauma, inflammatory disease and, in this context, surgery causing tissue damage. The latter results in the release of chemicals, some of which are responsible for the sensation of pain, for example substance-P, bradykinin and prostaglandin-E (Carr and Mann, 2000).

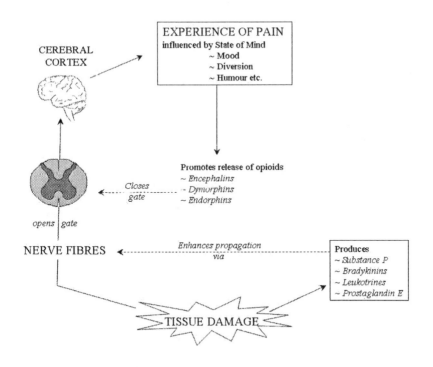

Cartoon 2.3: The physiological experience of pain

This physiological response begins with sensory neurones or nerve cells which detect the tissue damage and respond by relaying messages to the central nervous system. These nerve cells, which can be a metre long (Wood *et al*, 2004), 'fire', which means that information from the nerve ending travels along the myelinated axon by waves of electrical energy and carries the message from the receptor to the main part of the cell.

In turn, the message is then passed to nearby cells with the help of neurotransmitters. The myelin sheath is especially useful here in the conduction of nerve impulses (see *Cartoon 2.4*). This sensory information is then carried through electrical impulses to the spinal cord from any part of the body and will cause the sensation of pain. However, this will only happen if the intensity of injury-causing stimuli (otherwise known as noxious stimuli) is sufficient to cause, or to potentially cause, harm to the body.

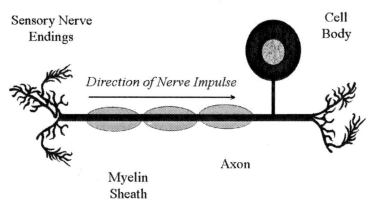

Cartoon 2.4: A sensory neurone

Nerve cells

These consist of one of three types: the A-delta and C-fibres responsible for carrying pain sensation, and the A-beta nerve fibres which are responsible for the non-painful sensations, eg. touch or temperature. The A-delta fibres will, when stimulated, carry the pain sensation quickly and cause an instantaneous reflex response provoking an immediate withdrawal of tissue from the damage source. So, as unpleasant as it is, pain does have a fundamental role in our survival.

Interestingly, these fibres are responsible for the 'first' or 'fast' pain sensation. This pain sensation is described as sharp and localised and continues to remain intact, serving as a protective barrier so that tissue is not further exposed to damage. So it is possible even for a patient who has had morphine postoperatively to feel pain sensation, eg. a pin prick, despite their initial post-operative pain being brought under control.

The C-fibres, in contrast to A-delta fibres, will transmit impulses at a slower rate and are referred to as the 'second pain' and described as a dull throbbing ache which is usually felt after the initial sharp pain. Finally, the A-beta fibres are usually activated by touch and sensation and are therefore not involved in the transmission of painful stimuli.

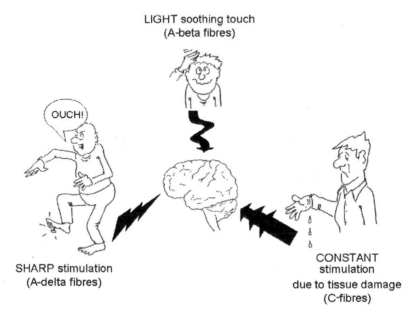

Cartoon 2.5: The action of A-delta, A-beta and C-fibres

Types of pain

The fact that there are a wide variety of pain sensations can be explained by the numerous causes of pain as well as the way we all react differently to painful stimuli which, to some extent, will determine the acuity or chronicity of pain (Kazanowski and Laccetti, 2002). The main types of pain are as follows:

Superficial

This is the result of localised superficial nerve cells which are stimulated in cutaneous tissue, eg. skin, and can result from mechanical injury, eg. scraping or compression, thermal or chemical injury.

Visceral (organ pain)

The nerve cells here are deeper and usually located in the thoracic, abdominal, pelvic or cranial cavities. This type of pain can also be 'referred' to other areas of the body and this means that, although the sensation comes from one organ or area of the body, it is perceived by the individual in another area.

Somatic (structural pain)

Pain is experienced as a result of a trauma or injury in muscles, joints, bones, ligaments, tendons and fascia and can be sharp and severe, or dull and achy, over a constant or intermittent period.

Pain as a result of metabolic need or excess

This is the result of vascular disease or vascular compromise, eg. atherosclerosis. In arterial vascular disease, ischaemic pain is experienced due to insufficient oxygen and nutrients. Pain can also be the result of an aneurysm in which blood flow is restricted beyond it. Similarly, coronary artery disease is a narrowing of the coronary arteries compromising blood flow to the coronary muscle and will cause severe angina pain radiating to the left arm or jaw and giving a sense of 'crushing' pressure. By contrast, peripheral arterial disease is due to restricted circulation caused by hypovolaemia, blood clots or trauma, and results in a localised severe pain. Chronic peripheral arterial disease is a progressive narrowing of the peripheral arteries and arterioles and causes severe intermittent claudication.

Neuropathic pain

This results from damage to the peripheral or central nervous system and can be mild to severe and described as a 'burning' sensation. For example, phantom limb pain is an example of neuropathic pain and is pain experienced in the very part of the body which has been removed as a result of damaged nerves at the site of the stump. Since more than 90 per cent of amputees experience this problem, this suggests that pain is determined as much by the brain's abstract representation or map of the body as the condition of the body itself (Broks, 2004).

The nature and complexity of pain

The discussion so far has established that peripheral nerve fibres do respond to tissue damage and are able to convert mechanical, chemical and thermal stimuli into electrical signals which are sent to the spinal cord, then the brain stem and finally the brain. However, have you ever considered why some people, after having the same day surgery procedure, seem to feel pain more than others or why some people can experience excruciating pain when there is no apparent injury or, when there is a severe injury, the person may not feel any pain at all? The answers to these questions are found in seminal work during the 1960s by Patrick Wall, a neuro-physiologist and

Ronald Melzack, a psychologist. They proposed that there are powerful inhibitory or 'dampening influences' deep within the brain which send messages down the spinal cord and are able to close off the sensation of pain on entering the spinal cord and brain stem. The 'Melzack-Wall Gate Control Theory' (Melzack and Wall, 1965) had finally dispelled the long-standing theory (dating back to the philosopher Descartes) which argued that the intensity of pain was determined solely by the extent of tissue damage and was carried in one direction only from the site of damage to the brain.

The Melzack-Wall Gate Control Theory had established that the stimulation was being 'modulated', which means that the central nervous system was able to control the upstream flow of information to the brain. A little earlier we talked about chemicals which cause pain. By the same token, the body also produces opioid-like substances that can reduce the perception of pain and are called endogenous opioids (see *Cartoon 2.3*). Indeed without this controlling mechanism, the overload of sensory inputs may even cause epileptic fits (Fitzgerald, 2004). Thus the crux of the Gate Control Theory is one of central control in which cognitive or higher centres of the brain influence the perception of pain through fibres descending to the gating system and the ability to close this gate through cognitive activities such as distraction and relaxation. By contrast, activities such as anxiety and excitement will, in turn, open the gate resulting in an increased perception of pain (see *Cartoon 2.6*). This important work supports the idea that pain is a multidimensional experience of physical, psychological and social components.

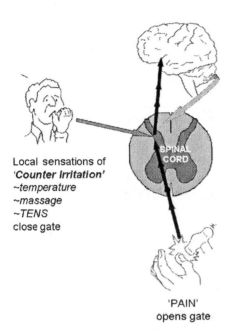

HIGHER CENTRE
INHIBITION
*e.g. mental state
distraction, humour
have an influence on
closing and keeping
the gate closed*

Local sensations of
'Counter Irritation'
~temperature
~massage
~TENS
close gate

'PAIN'
opens gate

Cartoon 2.6: The Gate Control Theory

Let us now look further at these other dimensions and understand a little more about how an integrated 'bio-psychological' approach can better explain the pain phenomenon.

Sensory dimension

This dimension represents pain in relation to its location (which part of the body), intensity (pain perception) and quality (how it feels). As you will see later, the intensity of pain is an individual experience and an important factor which needs to be assessed and managed. This is especially important within the day surgery context where patient stays are short and the need to maintain effective pain control before and after discharge is paramount. More information on the assessment of pain can be found on page 75.

Affective dimension

This focuses on the emotional response to pain and can be both a cause and consequence of it (Hawthorn and Redmond, 1998). Such emotional responses could include depression, anxiety, anger, agitation, mood changes, anticipation and irritability. For example, Broks (2004: p1), a neuropsychologist, describes how a patient of his complained of

> '...thumping headaches, excruciating stomach cramps, sore feet, sharp stabs at the small of his back and burning, tingling fingers.'

It was soon discovered that these very real physical symptoms of pain were in fact resulting from the grief he was experiencing on the anniversary of his son's death.

Cognitive dimension

The word cognitive suggests that the individual's thought processes will influence the perception of pain. This involves how individuals perceive themselves, what pain means to them and how they cope with it, as well as their attitudes and beliefs about it. Knowledge about pain is also important here. I am sure you will agree that the more informed you are about something, whether it be obtaining a mortgage or buying a car, the less threatening the experience will be. Well, this scenario is similar to that of undergoing a day surgery operation. Important work by Hayward (1975) and Boore (1978), and more recently by Barthelsson et al (2003a;b), Dewar et al (2003) and Skilton (2003) argues that patients who are well prepared for their surgery are less anxious and experience less pain.

Behavioural dimension

When people experience pain, they will normally demonstrate a variety of different observable behaviours, all of which indicate that they are in pain. These may include: verbalisation or vocalisation, eg. crying, moaning or sobbing; body movements, eg. limping, immobilisation, restlessness or supporting the painful body parts; or facial expressions such as facial grimacing, clenched teeth and closed eyes. Some people adopt pain control related behaviours such as physical activity/inactivity, taking medications, sleeping, reading or watching television to take their minds off their pain.

Socio-cultural dimension

Have you ever thought about why people express their pain in different ways? Well, we now know that pain is not just a physiological response but will also include emotional and behavioural responses based on past experiences and perceptions of pain. I can recall, when I worked in the recovery unit, that whenever there was a laparoscopic sterilisation list, patients from Mediterranean, Indian and African countries seemed to verbalise their pain more than their Caucasian counterparts (see also Weissman *et al*, 2002). So pain will also exist as part of the individual's demographic, ethnic, cultural, spiritual, religious and social world.

> *'Unless one listens to the patient's story and places it within the context of his thoughts, beliefs and culture, the patient's symptoms and responses (or lack thereof) to treatment cannot be understood.'*
>
> (Loeser, 2004: 12)

Implications for pain assessment

Now that the phenomenon of pain as a multidimensional concept has been introduced, its multidimensional nature will be of great importance when it comes to assessing the day surgery patient's pain. The assessment of pain is important as it allows us to gather data to help reduce the patient's pain to what I would describe as an 'acceptable' level. Although it is unrealistic for a patient not to expect to have pain after day surgery, by the same token, it would be unacceptable for a patient to experience a severe level of pain, particularly on their return home. Thus, the main purpose of pain assessment is to identify those patients who have pain and are at risk of developing it, as well as obtaining a baseline of information that will help us to decide on the most effective intervention.

Choice of assessment tool

As qualified nurses, I am sure you have come across several different pain assessment tools which help us to collect objective data about a patient's pain and you may well be using one in your area of practice at the moment. Unfortunately, pain assessment tools are used infrequently in the clinical area and this issue is discussed further, in addition to the responsibility of the nurse in fulfilling the role of pain assessor, in Chapter 4. However, in selecting the most appropriate pain assessment tool, it is important to consider those dimensions of pain that need to be assessed. Although we know that all these dimensions are important, some may be irrelevant for specific conditions or populations.

When selecting the most appropriate pain assessment tool for a day surgery unit, to all intents and purposes, patients are 'healthy' and waiting for an elective routine surgical procedure. Furthermore, they have been pre-operatively assessed, have fulfilled the selection criteria and have been judged fit enough to have surgery and return home on the same day, provided that they have adequate social support. Other considerations would also involve a variation in age range, socio-economic status and education level. Therefore, it is important that a pain assessment tool is easy to understand, valid, reliable and able to incorporate the patient's perception of pain. Indeed, the most reliable indicator of pain is the person's own report of it. Another important consideration is the fact that the day surgery population is transient and will be in and out of the unit within hours. On that basis, it is the sensory dimension or intensity of their pain that we are interested in assessing. An assessment tool is therefore required which is quick to administer; after all, the nature of pain can change within minutes. So, we need to gain as much information about the severity of pain fairly quickly given that the patient is expected to return home within a few hours.

But what are the most suitable tools for a day surgery unit, which are able to meet these criteria? Pain assessment tools are broadly classified as single/unidimensional or multi-dimensional depending on how pain is measured. In the former, it is the intensity or severity of pain which is measured whereas the latter will include the intensity, location, duration, type and affective dimensions. Here is a small selection of some pain assessment tools which are used.

Table 2.1: Pain assessment tools

Uni-dimensional	Multi-dimensional
Verbal Descriptor/Rater Scale (VD/RS)	Pain Diary
	Pain Drawing
Numerical Rating Scale (NRS)	McGill Pain Questionnaire (MPQ)
Visual Analogue Scale (VAS)	and Short Form MPQ

Verbal Descriptor/Rater Scale (VD/RS)

This scale was developed by Keele (1948) and was originally based on three to five numerically ranked words such as

None   Slight   Mild   Moderate   Severe

These were used to assess responses to analgesia over a 24-hour period. Since then, the scale has been a very popular choice of pain assessment measurement. Twenty years later, Melzack and Casey (1968) used a modified VDS as part of the McGill Pain Questionnaire (MPQ) which was a five-point scale using an intensity range from 'no pain' through to 'excruciating'.

Advantages and disadvantages

This scale has been described as simple to complete and usable for patients with chronic and acute pain (Flaherty, 1996). However, the scale does restrict patients to indicating the intensity of their pain by selecting one word only, although this may not necessarily reflect their interpretation of it (Flaherty, 1996; McGuire, 1988). There is also the potential for ambiguity in some of the words used. For example, 'mild' to one patient may mean 'slight' pain to another. Furthermore, the severity of pain can also be confused with its frequency. For example, pain may be severe but not experienced very often. Someone may therefore describe their pain as mild.

Numerical Rating Scale (NRS)

This scale can be described as either a horizontal or vertical line with zero '0' indicating no pain located at the bottom or one extremity and '4' indicating severe pain at the top, and is a popular choice amongst researchers (Heron and Lozinguez, 1999; Jensen *et al*, 2001)

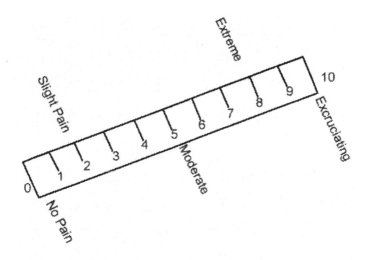

Pain Ruler

Cartoon 2.7: The Numerical Rating Scale

Although the NRS was originally published as a line with the scale of 0–10, there are currently multiple versions of it, all of which try to improve its ease of administration and scoring (Flaherty, 1996).

Advantages and disadvantages

The main advantages of the NRS are its simplicity of administration, scoring and use, and the fact that it does not involve a need for knowledge of the English language. Unlike the VDS, there is no potential for ambiguity of words as numbers are used. However, it has been described as unreliable, particularly for the elderly or for very young patients who may not be able to differentiate between the numbers (for example, a rating of 5 will indicate a higher level of pain than 2) (Flaherty, 1996). Moreover, the NRS like the VDS has discrete categories in which the respondent must choose only one, thus there is an element of fixed choice.

Visual Analogue Scale (VAS)

This scale consists of a line, usually 100mm in length or occasionally 150 or 160mm (Price *et al*, 1983). The anchors at each of the end of the VAS line indicate extremes of the sensation being measured with the left side representing 'No pain' and the other end representing 'Worst possible pain'. The intensity of the sensation is scored by measuring the mms from the left hand (lower) end of the scale to the mark made by the respondent, thus a number between 0 and 100 will indicate the severity of pain.

No pain   Worst possible pain

Figure 2.3 Visual Analogue Scale—VAS

Advantages and disadvantages

The VAS has been described by Katz and Melzack (1999) as being easy and short to complete thus making it easy to administer and score, as well as it being simple to understand. Main reported criticisms have included the difficulty of administering it during the post-operative period due to the effects of the anaesthetic, nausea and blurred vision (DeLoach *et al*, 1998). Moreover, respondents with cognitive and motor problems (Carr and Mann, 2000) arising from conditions such as rheumatoid arthritis may also experience difficulty in completing the scale (Katz and Melzack, 1999).

Pain Diaries

This method of obtaining information about pain from the individual's own perspective can prove to be very useful in gaining more of an insight into those factors which may increase or decrease their pain.

Advantages and disadvantages

One of the main advantages of this method is that it enables patients to be more actively involved in the decision making about their care and it can be a useful source of information about the impact of pain on a person's life over time without the problem of recall bias. However, by contrast, the principle of having to record pain frequently in a diary may cause a patient to become almost obsessive about it and it may provide inaccurate information.

So far, the pain assessment tools discussed have been unidimensional scales in that the intensity or severity of pain only has been addressed. One of the main criticisms of these tools has been that it is difficult to convert a multidimensional sensation on a single scale. The next set of pain assessment tools reviewed are an attempt to redress this criticism.

Pain Drawing

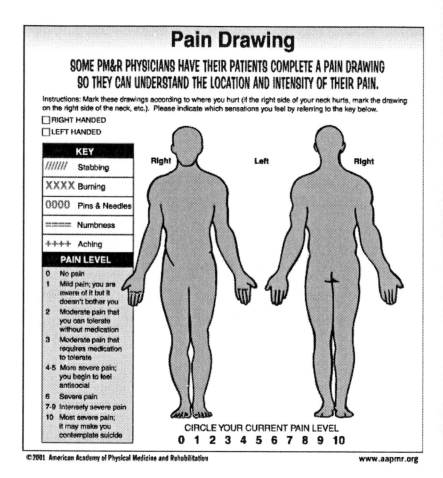

Figure 2.4: Pain Drawing (copyright American Academy of Physical Medicine and Rehabilitation)

This visual method of pain assessment is a quick and easy way of locating pain by asking the individual to indicate where their pain is as well as assessing its quality. A Pain Diagram is also included as part of the McGill Pain Questionnaire and the Wisconsin Brief Pain Questionnaire.

Wong-Baker FACES Pain Rating Scale

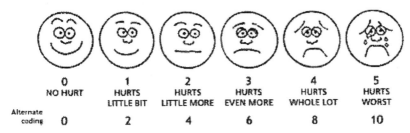

Figure 2.5: Wong-Baker FACES Pain Rating Scale
Reprinted by permission from Wong DL *et al* (2001)

This tool consists of faces ranging from a big smile to tears with associated numbers indicating pain intensity. This scale is particularly useful for children and cognitively impaired patients.

McGill Pain Questionnaire (MPQ)

This assessment tool allows measurement of several features of the pain experience including location, intensity and pattern over time. The scoring method includes the sensory, affective and evaluative dimensions of pain. The indices used are the Total Pain Rating Index (PRI-T), four sub-indices (PRI-sensory, PRI-affective, PRI-evaluative and PRI-miscellaneous), nine words chosen to describe the pain and the Present Pain Intensity (PPI).

McGill Pain Questionnaire

Patient's Name ____________ Date ________ Time ________ am/pm

PRI: S ______ (1-10) A ______ (11-15) E ______ (16) M ______ (17-20) PRI(T) ______ (1-20) PPI ______

1 FLICKERING QUIVERING PULSING THROBBING BEATING POUNDING	11 TIRING EXHAUSTING
2 JUMPING FLASHING SHOOTING	12 SICKENING SUFFOCATING
3 PRICKING BORING DRILLING STABBING LANCINATING	13 FEARFUL FRIGHTFUL TERRIFYING
4 SHARP CUTTING LACERATING	14 PUNISHING GRUELLING CRUEL VICIOUS KILLING
5 PINCHING PRESSING GNAWING CRAMPING CRUSHING	15 WRETCHED BLINDING
6 TUGGING PULLING WRENCHING	16 ANNOYING TROUBLESOME MISERABLE INTENSE UNBEARABLE
7 HOT BURNING SCALDING SEARING	17 SPREADING RADIATING PENETRATING PIERCING
8 TINGLING ITCHY SMARTING STINGING	18 TIGHT NUMB DRAWING SQUEEZING TEARING
9 DULL SORE HURTING ACHING HEAVY	19 COOL COLD FREEZING
10 TENDER TAUT RASPING SPLITTING	20 NAGGING NAUSEATING AGONIZING DREADFUL TORTURING
	PPI 0 NO PAIN 1 MILD 2 DISCOMFORTING 3 DISTRESSING 4 HORRIBLE 5 EXCRUCIATING

BRIEF MOMENTARY TRANSIENT	RHYTHMIC PERIODIC INTERMITTENT	CONTINUOUS STEADY CONSTANT

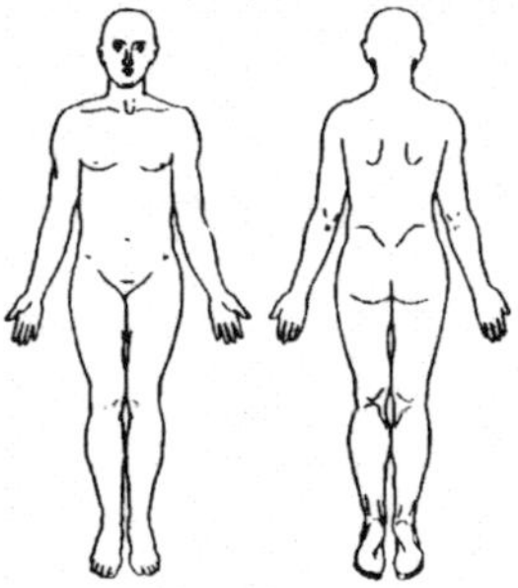

E = EXTERNAL

I = INTERNAL

COMMENTS:

FIG. 2. McGill Pain Questionnaire. The descriptors fall into four major groups: sensory, 1 to 10; affective, 11 to 15; evaluative, 16; and miscellaneous, 17 to 20. The rank value for each descriptor is based on its position in the word set. The sum of the rank values is the pain rating index (PRI). The present pain intensity (PPI) is based on a scale of 0 to 5. Copyright 1970 Ronald Melzack.

Figure 2.6 McGill Pain Questionnaire reprinted by permission of Melzack, R

Advantages and disadvantages

A principal recommendation for this scale is the number of studies supporting its reliability and validity (Byrne et al, 1982; Graham et al, 1980; Klepac et al, 1981; McGuire, 1984; Prieto et al, 1980). Not only can this tool be successfully used in obtaining data on qualitative and quantitative aspects of pain, it also addresses the multidimensionality of it (Flaherty, 1996). It is also widely used with approximately 24 translations in fifteen languages (Van Duijn, 1995). However, one of its main disadvantages is that it is demanding on patients and requires up to 30 minutes to complete (Flaherty, 1996; McGuire, 1988).

Although there is now a shorter version (SF-MPQ), this tool has been less investigated psychometrically. As with any attempt to measure a subjective experience using words, it is also possible that patients might not understand the adopted descriptions of pain. For example, Padfield (2004) reports on a recent experiment in which a group of people were asked to hold their hand in a cup of ice for one minute. The group were then asked to rate their experience using SF-MPQ. It was found that the sensation people experienced not only ranged in quality, but also produced different ranges of intensity from 1 to 9 on the VAS. It is evident therefore that the same experience produced a variation of responses.

Which assessment tool is suitable for a day surgery unit?

From the discussion so far, the VDS has been argued to be unsuitable within the day surgery context on the grounds of interpretability. This is because of the ambiguity of the verbal descriptors used and the fact that the respondents can choose one word only from a collection of words which may not adequately reflect their experience of pain. This restriction may also limit the acceptability of the scale. In the case of NRS, this numerical tool also has discrete response options and the respondent chooses one integer only, thus its acceptability and preciseness can be questioned. There is also potential for the scale to be unreliable, as some respondents may not be able to differentiate between the numbers, which may also limit its interpretability. It is also difficult for the MPQ to be used for a day surgery population since it can take up to 30 minutes to complete. Even when the short form version of this tool is used, given the transient nature of the day surgery stay, it will be more appropriate to measure the intensity of pain rather than its duration and pattern over time.

Of the pain assessment tools briefly reviewed, the VAS arguably rates as the best (Coll *et al*, 2004a). Not only does it have methodological qualities of reliability (it is consistent), validity (it is measuring what it is supposed to be measuring), sensitivity (it can measure small differences between the scores) and appropriateness for a day surgery population, it is also one of the most widely used assessment tools for post-operative pain (Briggs and Dean, 1998; Gudex *et al*, 1996). The use of the VAS as a pain measurement tool benefits the respondent, as it uses few words so vocabulary is less of an issue (Flaherty, 1996). Indeed, provided that clear instructions are given to the respondent, it is reasonably simple to complete. Moreover, for the nurse assessing pain, it is easy and brief to administer and score (Katz and Melzack, 1999). It is also a good method of expressing pain severity (Huskisson, 1982; Scott and Huskisson, 1976). The VAS is like a measurement of weight in that there is a true zero point. Thus, differences between the VAS measurement can then be interpreted as meaningful percentages (Flaherty, 1996) and allow rigorous statistical tests to be conducted on average pain levels. Finally, there is the argument that the VAS is more sensitive than the NRS as it can both underestimate and overestimate pain in comparison with the VAS estimates. For example, the underestimated NRS score occurs by rounding down 34.9 mm to 3 on the NRS.

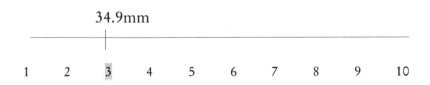

Figure 2.7: Overestimation of pain

Overestimation occurs by rounding up a VAS score of 35.0mm to 4 on the NRS. This means that a difference of 0.1 mm between the VAS scores would constitute a whole integer difference on the NRS.

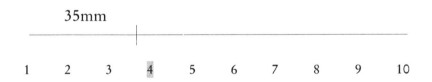

Figure 2.8: Underestimation of pain

Furthermore, the VAS continues to be cited in much of the contemporary literature on pain as the main assessment tool (Chung *et al*, 2001; Good, 1999; Kelly, 2000; Marquie *et al*, 2003; Quigley *et al*, 2002; Sjostrom *et al*, 2000,). Thus the availability of a unified and reliable measure of pain such as the VAS can address its sensory dimension and will provide reliable information about the intensity of pain.

Summary

In this chapter, pain has been defined as a complex concept comprising of several dimensions. The 'total' pain experience was considered as well as how pain will affect the individual physically, psychologically and socially. These dimensions were then discussed in more detail. The physical/physiological dimension considered the role of nociceptors as well as A-delta, A-beta and C-fibres and the different types of pain. The psychological/affective/cognitive dimensions were then presented, as well as the social/socio-cultural dimension and their importance in influencing pain perception. The latter half of the chapter focused on the importance of pain assessment followed by a review of both uni- and multidimensional pain assessment tools with the argument for using the VAS as the most appropriate tool within the day surgery context.

The next chapter presents some of the research on pain experience after day surgery.

Further reading

Coll AM, Ameen J, Mead D (2004a) Postoperative pain assessment tools in day surgery: a critical review. *J Adv Nurs* 46(2): 124–33

Coll AM, Ameen J, Moseley L (2004b) A critical review of reported pain after day surgery. *J Adv Nurs* 46(1): 53–65

Coll AM, Ameen J (2005) Profiles of pain after day surgery: Patients' experiences of three different operation types. *J Adv Nurs* (in press)

Coll AM, Ameen J (2004) Zeneca Travelling Fellowship Report: Day surgery discharge policies in Australia. *J One Day Surgery* Feb: 18–21

Davis P (1993) Opening up the Gate Control Theory. *Nurs Stan* 7(45): 25–27

McCaffery M (1989) *Pain: Clinical Manual for Nursing Practice*, 2nd edn. Mosby, St. Louis

Melzack R, Wall PD (2004) *The Challenge of Pain*, 2nd edn. Penguin Global, London

Wall PD, Melzack R, eds (1999) *Textbook of Pain*, 4th edn. Churchill Livingstone, London

3

What does the research say on pain after day surgery?

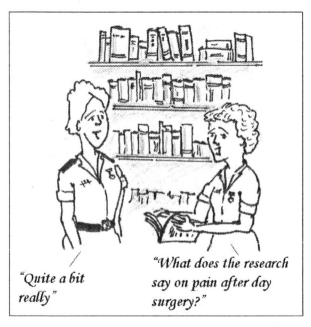

"Quite a bit really"

"What does the research say on pain after day surgery?"

Cartoon 3.1: What does research say on pain after day surgery?

Learning outcomes

At the end of this chapter, the nurse will:

- Be able to understand the misconception of the pain experience after day surgery;
- Have a comprehensive knowledge of reported pain after day surgery;

37

- Understand the inconsistencies in the literature in reporting pain after day surgery; and
- Appreciate the need for a greater consistency of pain reporting.

Introduction

During an interview of twenty laparoscopic sterilisation patients, it was clear that severe pain was experienced.
   '..But when I went down and came round, I remember waking up and thinking how much it hurt. Em, I was surprised. I wasn't led to believe it would hurt as much as it did.'
(Patient B)

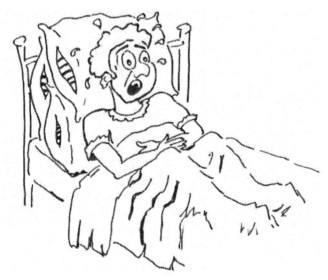

"I wasn't led to believe it would hurt as much as it did"

Cartoon 3.2: A patient in pain

How often have patients told you this? It is certainly not uncommon for patients to be surprised by the severity of the pain they have experienced after day surgery. This severity is well documented in the literature and forms the focus of this chapter.

Misconceptions of pain experience

Given the vast improvements in surgical techniques, anaesthesia and analgesia over the last 25 years, you (the healthcare professional) might believe that:

- Pain after day surgery should be minimal; and

- Recent evidence (post 1990) suggests that there is a lower incidence and lower severity of pain than studies from an earlier period.

Unfortunately, you would be wrong on both counts. As you will see, pain experience after day surgery continues to be at a severe level, even for the most common procedures. The more recent studies do not show lower levels of pain than the earlier ones, which is rather unexpected. It also seems to be the case that patients and their relatives do tend to equate day surgery

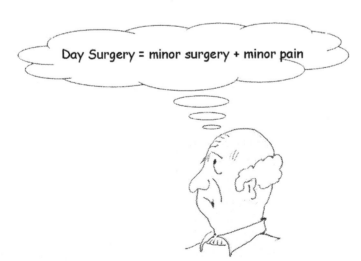

Cartoon 3.3: Day surgery equation

with minor surgery and minor pain experience afterwards as the quotation above suggests (Thatcher, 1996).

Consequently, the severe level of pain experience comes as a nasty surprise when patients are not able to return to work as soon as they had planned and need extra support at home to look after the children, housework, cooking etc. Indeed, within day surgery, this misconception is important both clinically and financially. We know from seminal work carried out (Boore, 1978; Hayward, 1975) that if patients are not informed and prepared for their surgery, they are likely to be more anxious, experience more pain and take longer to recover, with the potential for other complications to develop. There are also financial implications in terms of extra time taken off work, unplanned GP visits, extra prescription charges or even readmission to hospital. So what does the evidence say on pain experience after day surgery?

The evidence

Fifteen years ago, the Royal College of Surgeons and College of Anaesthetists (1990) stated that there was a high incidence of post-operative pain, with as many as three quarters of patients experiencing moderate to severe pain while in hospital. A year later, Firth (1991) found that between 63 and 100 per cent of day surgery patients were experiencing 'unacceptable' levels of pain during the first 24 to 48 hours following discharge. Wilkinson *et al* (1992), in their postal survey of 588 day surgery patients, found that patients were still experiencing pain on the second post-operative day. In 1994, a study by Oberle *et al* (1994) established that 36 per cent had continued to experience severe pain on the third post-operative day which they had not anticipated. These patients had undergone a range of minor and major day surgical procedures including arthroscopy, bunionectomy, cataract extraction and laparoscopic sterilisation. In Leith *et al*'s (1994) study, it was found that, although 91 per cent of day surgery units (n=147) had a protocol for the administration of analgesia to take home, pain was not controlled in two thirds (67 per cent) of the units examined.

More recently, Chung *et al* (1997) looked at the pain experience of patients who had undergone a range of day surgery orthopaedic, urological, general, ear, nose and throat (ENT), gynaecological and ophthalmic surgery in which five per cent of these patients (n=10,008) experienced severe pain on the first post-operative day. In 1998, Beauregard *et al* (1998) investigated pain experience after laparoscopy, knee or shoulder arthroscopy and carpal tunnel decompression (n=93). In this study, a numerical rating scale was used to assess pain severity at 24 and 48 hours and seven days post-operatively. Given that a numerical rating score of 4 or more was interpreted as 'moderate to severe' pain, at 24 hours 60 per cent rated their pain at this level. At 48 hours, 76 per cent experienced this level of pain.

What do you think was the patients' level of pain a week later?

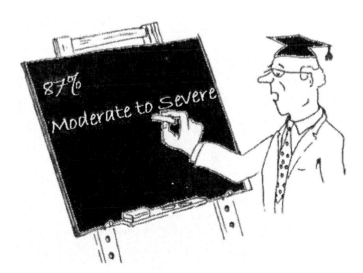

Cartoon 3.4: Level of pain experience

Surprisingly, 87 per cent of patients had rated their pain at a 'moderate to severe' level which is high and provides evidence of the severity of pain even a week after surgery.

A study by Agboola et al (1999) investigated pain experience for a sample of patients (n=40) who had undergone laparoscopic sterilisation. In this study, it was found that 65 per cent continued to experience a 'considerable amount of pain' on the third post-operative day. However, on the seventh post-operative day, 30 per cent were still 'in pain'. Two years later, a study by De Beer and Ravalia (2001) using a verbal descriptor scale showed that 34 per cent of laparoscopic sterilisation patients (n=100) had experienced moderate to severe pain on the day of surgery. In 2002, using the same method of data collection and the same operation type, Burumdayal and MacGowan-Palmer found that 55 per cent of patients had experienced moderate to severe pain.

In the case of laparoscopic sterilisation, it appears that severe pain is more likely to be experienced on the day of the operation and the first day afterwards. This is well documented in the literature (Chung et al, 1997; Lewin and Razis, 1995; Mackintosh and Bowles, 1998; Oberle et al, 1994; Westman et al 1996a; b). The severity of pain can be explained by the insertion of carbon dioxide gas into the abdomen and ischaemia of the fallopian tubes once they are ligated or occluded (Agboola et al, 1999).

In your own clinical areas, I am sure that the number of laparoscopic cholecystectomies is increasing. Based on a sample of 22 patients, a study by Parlow et al (1999) reported 'moderate to severe' pain on the day of surgery for 80 per cent of these patients. By noon the next day, the percentage experiencing pain at this level had decreased by almost half to 48 per cent. Khan et al (2002) specifically investigated a sample of 32 patients who had undergone this procedure using an 11-point numerical rating scale (0 to 10) and found that on the first post-operative day, a median score of 5 out of 10 was indicated as 'worst' pain. On day three, a median score of two out of ten was experienced as 'pain' which continued to day seven.

A more recent study by Watt-Watson *et al* (2004) found that patients who had undergone day surgery to their shoulder (n=48) had significantly more pain than those who had undergone laparoscopic cholecystectomy (n=54) or hand surgery (n=78). Similar to the latter study, pain was reported as 'moderate to severe'. In this study, the Brief Pain Inventory—Short-Form (BPI-SF) was used in a telephone interview at 24, 48 and 72 hours and seven days after discharge. This is an established multidimensional scale which measures the severity of pain and its impact on functioning (Cleeland and Syrjala, 1992).

From the literature so far, it is clear that significant levels of pain are experienced after day surgery. So, what is a realistic expectation of pain?

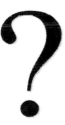

Cartoon 3.5

The expectation of pain

Do you think it is fair to assume that patients should return home after day surgery experiencing an element of pain or should they expect to be in a pain-free state? What is a realistic expectation? Many studies cited in the literature have referred to 'adequate pain relief' (Joshi, 1994), 'effectively treating post-operative pain' (White, 1995) and 'pain management' (Tong and Chung, 1999). Phrases such as these indicate that it is unlikely that patients will experience zero levels of pain, but that the pain they do experience can be brought to a low level by modern advances in the use of analgesia.

However, an agreed level in which pain should be regarded as unacceptable needs to be established. This is important because the established level of unacceptability should influence the nature and timing of giving analgesias. Indeed, several authors have tried to indicate what they consider to be morally unacceptable. Leith *et al* (1994) contends that no patient should expect more than 'moderate' pain. Lloyd and McLauchlan (1994) contend that post-operative pain should be kept to a 'minimal' level so that the patient should not suffer. Hitchcock and Ogg (1995) went further in stating that a pain-free state was possible. It was their opinion that patients should not only wake up safely after their anaesthetic, but also pain free. Tong and Chung (1999) contend that pain should be controlled to the extent that the patient can resume normal activities. These claims are important in providing the benchmark for an acceptable level of pain experience.

Yet it is unrealistic to expect no pain. However, a level of pain which is considered 'acceptable' remains unclear because there is a diversity in reported levels of pain after day surgery (Coll *et al*, 2004b). From the literature, it seems that pain intensity during day three is as severe as that reported on the day of surgery. It is possible that this is the result of differences in reported levels of pain by type of surgery, data collection methods, incidence and description of pain. Furthermore, the reliability and validity of these studies, as well as the method of sampling of patients, are questionable. It is also the case that differences relating to surgical speciality and operation type have not been addressed. I am sure you will agree that even within one surgical speciality, two surgical procedures are likely to result in two different reported levels of pain. For example, within the surgical speciality of gynaecology, laparoscopic sterilisation involves high levels of pain (as discussed earlier) and diagnostic laparoscopy is likely to involve moderate pain due to insufflation of carbon dioxide gas and associated trapped air (Agboola *et al*, 1999). By contrast, a dilatation and curettage generally causes a low level of pain (Petticrew *et al*, 1995).

When some studies state the operation type and others only state the speciality, it is difficult to obtain reliable estimates of the intensity of pain experienced for specific surgical operation types and to make recommendations on how healthcare professionals should prepare their patients. There is also the inconsistency in the use of descriptors for pain in these studies. For example, Oberle *et al* (1994) use the word 'severe' to describe pain related to specific operation types on the day of surgery while Jackson *et al* (1997) describe 'moderate to severe muscular pain' in relation to the surgical speciality on the day after surgery. This inconsistency also exists in descriptors of post-operative pain both across and within specific operation types. For example, Oberle *et al* (1994) report a nine per cent incidence of 'severe' pain on day three for patients undergoing laparoscopic sterilisation while Agboola *et al* (1999) report a 65 per cent incidence of 'considerable' pain on day three following the same operation type.

In a major research project that I conducted, one of the main objectives was to address these inconsistencies of pain reporting. The research was an investigation into the level of pain experience and the establishment of pain profiles for three of the most commonly performed operation types. Unsurprisingly, patients experienced severe pain as far as the third post-operative day.

At the time of conducting the study (Coll, 2001), there was little evidence to show the degree of impact of day surgery on patients' experiences. It was a national study which involved three day surgery units at three geographical locations in England and Wales and was based on operation types of hernia repair (inguinal, umbilical, para-umbilical and femoral), laparoscopic sterilisation and varicose veins (saphenous ligation, phlebectomies and avulsions). These operation types were also chosen as:

a) There was a 'high' or 'medium' likelihood of pain experience (Audit Commission, 1990);

b) They were more likely to have post-operative complications and symptoms when compared with other types of day surgery; and

c) Patients undergoing these procedures were more likely to have contact with the primary healthcare team after discharge.

It was designed as a pre- and post-operative postal survey sent out to 785 patients scheduled to have these procedures and included five health assessment tools used to provide a comprehensive health assessment of patients both before and after their surgery. The tools included SF36, Health Locus of Control, Satisfaction With Life, Duke UNC Functional Health Profile and the VAS which helped to capture the physiological, psychological and social dimensions of health. In total, 578 patients completed both the pre- and post-operative questionnaires giving a response rate of 79 per cent. In addition, semi-structured interviews were carried out on twenty patients selected from one centre who had undergone laparoscopic sterilisation to further support the findings, as it was found that patients undergoing this particular operation type were experiencing more severe pain on the day of surgery compared with the hernia and varicose vein patients. The main aims of the study were to:

• Investigate the pain experience of three commonly performed operation types as far as the third post-operative day using the VAS. In Chapter 2, we agreed that the VAS was found to be the most appropriate pain assessment tool for a day surgery population because of its reliability, validity and the fact that it is one of the most widely used pain assessment tools;

• Examine the intensity and duration of pain experience;

- Compare pain levels for three operation types; and
- Make recommendations for a day surgery unit discharge protocol based on the findings.

What level of pain on the VAS is acceptable?

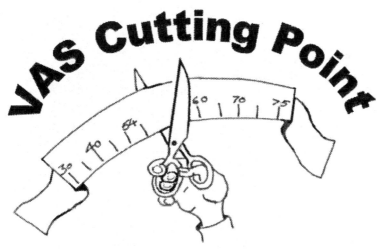

Cartoon 3.6: The VAS cutting point

An agreement on what level of pain is unacceptable will depend on what 'cutting point' is taken on the VAS. If we look to the literature for supporting evidence, it appears that, of those studies which have used the VAS in measuring pain experience and have indicated cutting points, few have justified them. The next table shows different authors' interpretations of what the VAS cutting point is, clearly demonstrating a difference in their judgements.

Table 3.1: A history of the VAS cutting points

Study	VAS cutting point
Seymour *et al* (1996)	>30mm
Westman *et al* (1996a)	>40mm
Westman *et al* (1996b)	>30–40mm (sic)
Collins *et al* (1997)	>54mm
Stubhaug *et al* (1995)	>60mm
Slappendel *et al* (1999)	>70mm
Curtis *et al* (1994)	>75mm

It was decided that the fairest method of undertaking an analysis of pain experience would be to use three different cutting points of 30, 40 and 50mm; any patient scoring below 30mm was experiencing minimal pain and any score of above 50mm indicated a severe level of pain, with differing levels of unacceptability between 30 to 50mm.

The findings

At this stage, it is useful to provide an overview of the likely level of pain that can be expected for each of the three operation types investigated in this research study:

- Hernia patients are likely to experience the most pain given that the incision is the largest of the three operation types and there is a need for a longer recovery (McMenemin, 1999);

- Laparoscopic sterilisation patients are most likely to experience severe pain on the day of surgery and first day post-operatively due to experiencing tubal ischaemia and the presence of carbon dioxide gas. It is probable that pain will decrease steadily thereafter (Agboola *et al*, 1999; Fraser *et al*, 1989); and

• Varicose vein patients are unlikely to experience uncontrolled symptoms, although episodes of aching and bruising are expected (Baccaglini et al, 1997; Hardman et al, 1995; Sanders, 1995).

The results presented in the following tables show the incidence of pain by the respective operation type at the three cutting points over four days.

Table 3.2: The incidence of pain (%) on the day using three cutting points on the VAS for all patients

	VAS level of 30mm (%)	VAS level of 40mm (%)	VAS level of 50mm (%)
On the day of surgery	59 (n=355)	52 (n=314)	42 (n=250)

Clearly, depending on which cutting point is taken, the level of unacceptable pain on the day could be as high as 59 per cent or as low as 42 per cent. Also, it should be noted that there is a degree of overlap between the three cutting points reported in *Table 3.2*. Thus the reported percentages will not add up to 100 per cent because of this overlap. This is the case as patients with 50mm cutting points will be suffering at 30 and 40mm cutting points as well. This is also the case with the figures reported in *Tables 3.3, 3.4* and *3.5*.

Table 3.3: Analyses of pain experience at the three cutting points over four days

	VAS level of 30mm (%)	VAS level of 40mm (%)	VAS level of 50mm (%)
On the day of surgery	59	52	41
First day post-operatively	60	50	39
2nd day post-operatively	54	43	32
3rd day post-operatively	44	35	25

Even three days after surgery, 44 per cent of patients still experienced pain at 30mm and above. At 50mm, 25 per cent of patients experienced a severe level of pain.

Table 3.4 The incidence of pain (%) on the day at each cutting point and by operation type

	Hernia (%)	Lap sterilisation (%)	Varicose veins (%)	Overall (%)
30mm	59	74	47	59
40mm	52	67	41	52
50mm	41	56	30	42
Total number	244	170	185	599

On the day of surgery, laparoscopic sterilisation patients experienced the highest level of pain at each of the three cutting points. At 30mm and above, three quarters of patients experienced pain. Even at 50mm and above, over half of these patients had severe levels of pain. It is also clear that laparoscopic sterilisation patients experienced the most pain overall.

Table 3.5: The incidence of pain (%) on the third day at each cutting point and by operation type

	Hernia (%)	Lap sterilisation (%)	Varicose veins (%)	Overall (%)
30mm	54	32	41	44
40mm	44	25	33	35
50mm	29	17	26	25
Total number	244	170	185	599

When pain experience was investigated on the third post-operative day, there is no doubt that significant levels of pain were experienced by patients. It is also the case that more hernia patients experienced pain at a severe level compared with the other operation types.

Are you surprised by these results?

Before the results, we predicted that hernia patients would experience significantly more pain compared with the other operation types under consideration due to the length of the incision made. Clearly, this was the case as over one third of patients experienced pain at 50mm and above on the third post-operative day.

We also predicted that laparoscopic sterilisation patients would be more likely to experience severe pain on the day and first day post-operatively due to tubal ischaemia experienced and the presence of carbon dioxide gas. Pain would then steadily decrease thereafter. It was found that these patients had significantly experienced the highest level of pain on the day of surgery (56%) compared to the other operation types although hernia patients had the highest level of pain on the first post-operative day (44%) and third post-operative day (29%) compared with 26 per cent for the varicose vein patients.

Finally, varicose vein patients were predicted not to experience uncontrolled symptoms, although episodes of aching and bruising were expected. However, this prediction has not been substantiated since it was found that one quarter of varicose vein patients significantly experienced pain at 50mm and above on the third post-operative day. This is rather surprising as the limited amount of literature available on this operation type does not report such high levels of pain (Baccaglini *et al*, 1997; Linden and Bergbom Engberg, 1995).

It appears, therefore, that these findings support the general consensus that severe levels of pain are experienced after day surgery.

Summary

In this chapter, the misconception of pain after day surgery has been introduced, as well as a review of pain reports after day surgery from the literature. The main inconsistencies in how it has been reported have also been presented. However, in spite of the inconsistencies reported in the literature, its prevalence and incidence are set to continue unless knowledge of pain assessment and the administration of analgesia are improved. The onus of responsibility should, to a large extent, be on the nurse, since the post-operative care and decision to discharge the patient is ultimately made by the nurse.

The next chapter looks more closely at who is responsible for pain relief and the problems of pain assessment and management within nursing.

Further reading

Coll AM, Ameen J (2005) Profiles of pain after day surgery: Patients' experiences of three different operation types. *J Adv Nurs* (in press)

Coll AM, Ameen J, Moseley L (2004b) Reported pain after day surgery: a critical literature review. *J Adv Nurs* 46(1): 53-65

James D (2000) Patient perceptions of day surgery. *Br J Periop Nurs* 10(9): 466–72

Mitchell, MJ (1999) Patients' perceptions of day surgery: a literature review. *Ambulatory Surg* 7(2): 65–67

Noah N (2003) *A Study of the Economic Impact of Day Surgery on Primary Care Services and the Social Impact on Patients.* Department of Health, London

4

Who is responsible?

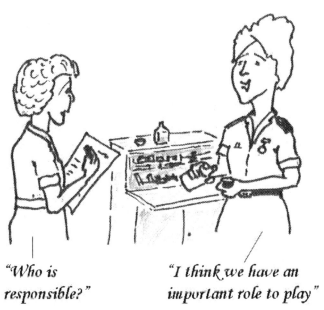

"*Who is responsible?*"   "*I think we have an important role to play*"

Cartoon 4.1: Who is responsible?

Learning outcomes

At the end of this chapter the nurse will:

- Understand that they can improve their skills in the assessment and management of pain;
- Have a comprehensive knowledge of the literature to support this argument;
- Understand the importance of their responsibility as the patient's advocate in assessing and managing pain; and

- Understand the need to constantly evaluate and update their pain assessment and management skills.

Introduction

Instances of acute post-operative pain are the most common clinical situations faced by day surgery nurses. However, from the literature, there is much evidence to suggest that both nurses and doctors lack knowledge about pain and the way it should be managed (De Rond et al, 1999; Schafheutle et al, 2001; Tanabe and Buschmann, 2000). From the medical perspective, it seems that doctors are failing to prescribe effective analgesia with little adherence to dosage protocols (Hawthorn and Redmond, 1998). It has also been suggested that the dose of opioids prescribed for patients is below therapeutic levels (Donovan et al, 1987; Marks and Sacher, 1973). McCaffery et al (1990) and Clarke et al (1996) make reference to inappropriate attitudes and beliefs held by both doctors and nurses, as well as poor monitoring of the patient's response to treatment.

> 'The nurse is one of the healthcare professionals who has frequent contact with patients receiving care in the community, at home or in in-patient or out-patient settings. This frequent contact puts the nurse in a unique position to identify the patient who has pain and its impact on the patient, patient's family and health professionals, to initiate action to alleviate the pain using available resources and to evaluate the effectiveness of those actions.'
>
> International Association for the Study of Pain, 1994: 2

Nurses do spend more time with patients and remain their advocate more than any other healthcare professional (Nash et al, 1999). It is the nurse who decides on the timing, administration route and dose of the drug to be given. The management of side effects is also important, so knowledge of the following is needed:

- How analgesia works;
- What the side effects are; and
- The dosages and frequency of use.

Ultimately, the nurse is responsible for identifying the physiological, psychological and social dimensions that will influence the patient's expression of pain. As we discussed in Chapter 2, the uniqueness of the pain experience is not only shaped by the individual's physical functioning but also by their:

- Emotions;
- Work;
- Family;
- Behaviours; and
- Socio-cultural background.

Thus it is the nurse's assessment of pain, determined by observational and interpersonal skills, which is essential to the post-operative recovery of the patient (Hawthorn and Redmond, 1998). It must be remembered that unrelieved pain is stressful for the patient and the nurse, so effective assessment of it is important (Emflorgo, 1999).

Could we do it better?

Since the 1970s, the nurse's role in the assessment and management of pain of the surgical patient has been a theme in the literature, and it seems that we can improve our pain assessment and management skills. The Report of The Working Party on Pain after Surgery for the Royal College of Surgeons and the College of Anaesthetists (1990) stated that nurses were lacking in the knowledge of, and commitment to, satisfactory post-operative pain control. Although this report was published fifteen years ago, the situation has changed very little. The literature suggests that there is a deficit in knowledge, but this is one of several barriers to effective pain control and is worthy of some discussion here.

Nurse barriers to effective pain management

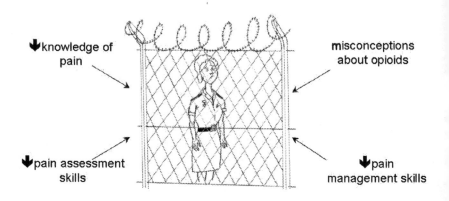

Cartoon 4.2: Nurse barriers to managing pain

Knowledge of pain

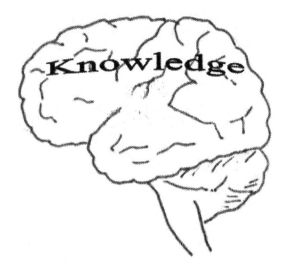

Cartoon 4.3: Knowledge of pain

It could be argued that due to the transience of day surgery patients and the speed at which they are discharged, nurses have restricted time for pre- and post-operative teaching about pain management. While this is true to some extent, it seems that nursing and medical curricula are failing to provide healthcare professionals with sufficient knowledge about:

- The multidimensional nature of pain and what causes it;
- The differences between chronic and acute pain;
- The effects of different factors on pain expression;
- Pain assessment methods;
- Pharmacology; and
- Pain management principles (Hawthorn and Redmond, 1998).

Also, few studies have been undertaken that look more closely at how pain education influences practice (Wallace *et al*, 1997: cited by Carr and Mann, 2000), as well as the lack of reporting on providing continuing professional education in pain management. Schafheutle *et al* (2001) maintain that nursing is frequently dominated by barriers of inaccurate and negative attitudes towards patients in pain, eg, patients experiencing acute post-operative pain can easily become addicted to opioids and should therefore not receive the full dose that they are entitled to. These attitudes are based on a combination of non-verbal cues, type of and time since surgery, and patient behaviour. The ward setting and policies such as workload and staff shortages have also added other barriers. From the literature, two themes seem to be apparent;

• Nurses underestimate patients' pain; and

• Nurses lack knowledge in the assessment and management of pain.

Pain assessment skills

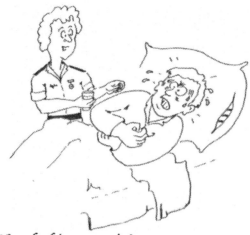

" *How bad is your pain?* "
" *Just try one for now ... see how it goes* "

Cartoon 4.4: Assessing pain

There has been much literature which suggests that nurses can do more to improve their pain assessment skills. There are several explanations why this may be the case. Firstly, nurses' perceptions of patients' pain are different; after all the experience of pain is unique for us all. It seems that nurses tend to overestimate the levels of least pain, underestimate the levels of worst pain and, as a result, overestimate the effectiveness of interventions used (Hawthorn and Redmond, 1998). This over- and underestimation occurs because nurses are making judgements about patients based solely on what they observe. There is also evidence that pain assessment tools are rarely used in practice (Hollingsworth, 1995: cited by Hawthorn and Redmond, 1998). Are you using a pain assessment tool in practice?

Nurses often make the assumption that patients will complain of pain; however, more often than not, patients expect the nurse to ask them about their pain (Seers, 1987). Even if an assessment of pain is made, it tends to be made during the medications round or, in the context here, when the day surgery patient first arrives back on the ward. A survey (n=180) of nurses conducted by Schafheutle *et al* (2001) found that nurses tended to rely on patients' non-verbal behaviour and used this to assess their analgesia requirements. A tendency to focus solely on the physical cause of pain without consideration of its multidimensional nature of emotional, spiritual and social factors, and incorrect interpretations of non-verbal cues, will generally result in a poor assessment. How often have you heard it said,

'Well, he can't be in that much pain because he is sleeping'?

Studies have shown that nurses have refused to believe what patients have said about their pain. Saxey (1986) found that 52 per cent of nurses did not believe the patient's report of it. This finding was also supported by a later study by Seers (1987). In a study by Brunier *et al* (1995), based on a pain survey of 514 qualified nurses, it was found that 27 per cent did not agree with the statement that they should believe the patient. Surprisingly, 44 per cent agreed with the statement that a doctor or a nurse's estimation of patients' pain should be regarded as being of more value than the patient's estimation!

A study by Mackintosh (1994) revealed that 72 per cent of nurses (n=44) did not feel confident in making 'accurate' assessments of patients' pain. It was also found that 87 per cent felt that they 'consistently' failed to estimate the level of pain patients experienced. In another study by Linden and Bergbom Engberg (1995), it was found that many nurses failed in reliably assessing pain when using both verbal and simple pain assessment tools. Zalon's study (1993) found that nurses (n=119) underassessed severe pain and over assessed mild pain. A study by Briggs and Dean (1998) compared transcripts of patient interviews (n=65) of their pain experience following elective orthopaedic surgery, with corresponding nursing records of these patient experiences. For example, the patient stated:

'My worst pain was last night. I am still in severe pain now'
(p 11)

By contrast, the nursing record indicated:

'Satisfactory post-operative evening, oral analgesia given for pain, appears to have slept well.'
(p 11)

It is evident that there is a clear difference between patients' and nurses' reports of the same situation.

The management of pain

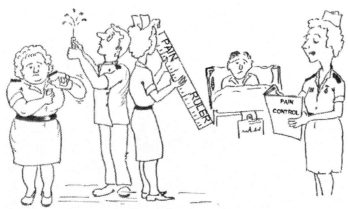

Now.... What shall we start with?
Cartoon 4.5: Managing pain

Not only is there evidence of nurses having a poor knowledge base of pain, there is evidence to suggest that there is also a poor knowledge base of pain management (Clarke *et al*, 1996;

De Rond *et al*, 1999; Tanabe and Buschmann, 2000). This is clearly demonstrated in a study by Brunier *et al* (1995), which focused on differences between chronic and acute pain. The study found that only seven per cent agreed with the statement that patients with severe chronic pain would need higher doses of analgesia than patients experiencing acute pain. It seems, therefore, that many nurses do not understand the difference between chronic and acute pain. In a US study by Tanabe and Buschmann (2000), a questionnaire on pain management principles for emergency nurses (n=1000) revealed deficits in knowledge on various pharmacologic analgesic principles. Nurses scored the lowest in the area of analgesics and their side effects, in which only 59 per cent of questions were answered correctly. Interestingly, these nurses did not understand the difference between physical dependence, addiction and tolerance, with only 61 per cent of questions answered correctly in this category. This is not surprising as it has recently been identified that, in the US, 78 per cent of all patients who attend A&E are in pain (Tanabe and Buschmann, 2000). In the UK, the figure is similar at 75 per cent (Audit Commission, 2001). It is also the case that nurses tend to under medicate patients when they administer only minimal amounts of analgesia (Nash *et al*, 1999). Lloyd and McLauchlan (1994), in their study of 269 trained nursing staff, found that an average of 25 per cent of nurses felt that patients should receive only minimal amounts of analgesia.

Poor documentation has also been suggested as a possible explanation for inadequate pain management. In a study by Tittle and McMillan (1994), it was found that documentation about pain was insufficient and that the effect of the medication was rarely recorded. In another study by Nash *et al* (1999), it was found that knowledge of documentation on pain assessment was limited. So it appears that information about patients' pain is often recorded inaccurately and, according to Hawthorn and Redmond (1998), poor documentation of pain may be a reflection of poor documentation in nursing generally.

Misconceptions about pain

Misconceptions compromise a nurse's ability to make optimal clinical decisions and have created an environment in which many ritualistic practices have dominated. There are several unfounded misconceptions about pain which need to be addressed here. The first misconception observed by many nurses relates to the fear of the patient becoming addicted to opioids. From my own experience as a day surgery recovery nurse, I have witnessed nurses who have administered small doses of an opioid analgesic to a patient in severe pain. They have decided not to administer the total amount the patient could have received because they were afraid that the patient would become addicted or would experience respiratory depression—two potential side effects after large doses of opioid analgesia. Fear of addiction or 'opiophobia' is a main reason for poor pain management and can result in nurses deliberately delaying the giving of analgesia or to administer less than the patient is entitled to, as my example demonstrates. This is a well-documented subject in the literature (Clarke *et al*, 1996; Nash *et al*, 1999).

Seers (1987) reported that 85 per cent of nurses (n=28) had overestimated the risk of patients becoming addicted to opioids. This finding also shows a lack of basic knowledge of the properties and actions of opioid analgesia (Hamilton and Edgar, 1992; McCaffery *et al*, 1990; Tanabe and Buschmann 2000; Yates *et al*, 1995). In a study by Clarke *et al* (1996) a survey of a 120 qualified nurses found that sixteen per cent believed that the incidence of addiction for patients treated with opioids was greater than 25 per cent. In fact, the actual incidence is known to be less than one per cent (Clarke *et al*, 1996). Tanabe and Buschmann (2000) found that only 28 per cent of emergency nurses were able to correctly identify this percentage.

Paradoxically, in another study it was found that nurses administered larger doses of opioid analgesics to males than to females during the initial post-operative period (McDonald, 1994). However, this practice is based on nothing more than folk belief since there is no scientific evidence to suggest that males should receive larger doses of opioids than females. In fact, there seems to be conflicting viewpoints in the literature. Some studies have reported that women report a higher incidence of pain than men (James *et al*, 1991; Kleinman, 1988; Lawlis *et al*, 1984). However, there is contrary evidence suggesting that more men suffer severe pain than women (Beauregard *et al*, 1998; Chung *et al*, 1997).

Of course, the fear of addiction is also closely linked with the fear of tolerance ie that the prolonged use of the analgesia will result in the body becoming used to the effects of it and no longer responding to the same extent. This is certainly more the case for terminally ill patients but still worthy of comment here. However, whether it is the case that a patient's tolerance is increasing or that their pain level is increasing due to the deterioration of their condition, it remains that very large doses of opioid analgesia can be given in order to control pain (Hawthorn and Redmond, 1998).

On a similar theme, the fear of respiratory depression is a common misconception yet it remains an uncommon side effect which is reversible by using Naloxone which is an opioid antagonist. It is also worth noting that the sensation of pain is a stimulus to respiration thus respiratory depression can only occur once pain is brought under control.

A further misconception is that of ageism based on beliefs that older patients have less pain sensitivity and increased tolerance of pain (Closs, 1996). As a result, opioids tend not to be administered because of fears of side effects and so pain remains uncontrolled. Given that the aging population is increasing and that chronological age is no longer an exclusion category for day surgery suitability, this issue requires further consideration as more elderly patients are likely to have day surgery in the future.

Patient barriers to effective pain management

Sometimes it is difficult for nurses to manage pain effectively

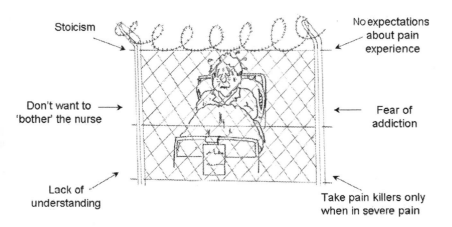

Stoicism

No expectations about pain experience

Don't want to 'bother' the nurse

Fear of addiction

Lack of understanding

Take pain killers only when in severe pain

Cartoon 4.6: Patient barriers to effective pain management

because of barriers patients bring to their encounters with healthcare professionals. Firstly, patients may be reluctant to trouble 'busy' nurses (Carr and Thomas, 1997). Some patients are fearful of being seen as not coping with their pain, as a nuisance and do not want to admit to being in pain (Carr, 1997). Other patients may feel that their pain is inevitable (Yates *et al*, 1995). This is particularly important if the patient has not been prepared for surgery and has no expectations about the likely level of pain to be experienced afterwards. Carr (1997) found that some patients would wait to be asked about their pain rather than volunteer the information.

Another important barrier is the patient's fear of becoming addicted to opioids (Tanabe and Buschmann, 2000). Scott and Hodson (1997: cited by Carr and Mann, 2000) found that almost 50 per cent of patients were prepared to suffer pain rather than complain about it. It is also possible that they may have had a bad experience with opioids on a previous occasion and experienced severe nausea and vomiting. As a result, they have decided to suffer the pain rather than experience the same symptoms.

Finally, possible reasons for why patients do not take their pain medication after their discharge home may be explained by the fact that patients do not understand how to take their analgesia, which could well be the result of poor information-giving by the nurse. It could also be because patients want to be 'in control' as the pain helps them to judge their level of activity. It may also be the caregivers who, because of their own fear of addiction or respiratory depression, may try to restrict the amount of analgesia taken by the patient (Hawthorn and Redmond, 1998).

While discussing the barriers to effective pain management, this chapter would not be complete without mentioning the organisational barriers which play an important role.

Organisational barriers to effective pain management

When I worked in the day surgery unit, it was before the introduction of under 24 hour surgery. Our unit closed at 6pm every evening. Thus, if we had concerns about a patient being discharged because of pain, it could be difficult to find a hospital bed in the main hospital, particularly if the hospital was on emergency intake. It was also the case that the patient was always keen to go home. On these occasions my concern was that if pain was uncontrolled before discharge, the patient's condition could deteriorate on their return home. Indeed, I often wondered what happened to these patients once they left us and this was one of the main incentives in carrying out my doctoral research.

Other organisational barriers include those of prescribing inappropriate and ineffective analgesia for operation types or, as my research showed, either not prescribing any medication to take home or charging patients for them. Finally, there are inconsistencies in the decision-making about which patients should receive a district nurse visit or, at least, a telephone call. This is a particular problem given the present nurse workforce shortages.

We can make it better—after all, it is our duty!

So far, we have learned that, although nurses play an important role in the assessment and management of patients' post-operative pain, a lot more can be done to improve this practice. Moreover, keeping up to date with new developments in analgesia and alternative therapies is in the NMC Code of Conduct:

> 'You have a responsibility to deliver care based on current evidence, best practice and, where applicable, validated research when it is available.'
>
> (NMC, 2002: 6.5: p8)

By keeping up to date, we will also be acting in our patients' best interests:

> 'You have a duty of care to your patients and clients who are entitled to receive safe and competent care.'
>
> (NMC, 2002: 1.4: p3)

Quite simply, unless we are adhering to these guidelines, how can we say that we are competent to assess and manage our patients' pain?

Summary

In this chapter, we have looked at who is responsible for the severe levels of pain which continue to be experienced after day surgery. The main barriers to effective pain assessment and management were categorised into nurse, patient and organisational barriers. In the nursing section, the main problems that have been highlighted so far have included a deficit in knowledge about pain and its management, the lack of use of pain assessment tools and differences in the way pain is perceived by the nurse and the patient, inadequate documentation and fear of addiction to opioids.

It appears that there is a lack of knowledge about pain and how to effectively manage it, since nurses do not always utilise research findings in their practice (Default *et al*, 1995: cited by Hawthorn and Redmond, 1998). From my own experience of teaching research methods, I am only too aware that student nurses not only have a negative attitude to research generally, but are also lacking the skills of how to interpret research findings. This problem continues to pose a challenge for lecturers who teach research skills.

Given the evidence, nurses do play a pivotal role in the care of the post-operative patient. After all, they spend most of their time with the patient and have a responsibility for ensuring that their pain assessment and management skills are evidence-based. Ultimately, they are the ones who will take the decision to discharge once the patient has been fully informed and has received appropriate analgesia to take when recovering at home.

In the next chapter, 'How can I make it better?' recommendations are made for how the situation can be redressed.

Further reading

Cohen FL (1980) Post surgical pain relief : patients' status and nurses' medication choices. *Pain* **9**: 265–74

Jackson IRB (2001) The management of pain following day surgery. *Br J Anaesthesia* (CEPD) **1**(2): 48–51

McCaffery M, Beebe A (1994) *Pain: Clinical Manual for Nursing Practice.* CV Mosby, London

McCaffery M, Ferrell BR (1997) Nurses' knowledge of pain assessment and management: how much progress have we made? *J Pain Symptom Man* **14**: 175–88

5

How can I make it better?

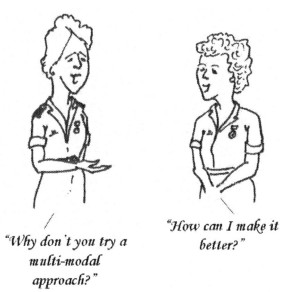

"Why don't you try a multi-modal approach?"

"How can I make it better?"

Cartoon 5.1: How can I make it better?

Learning outcomes

At the end of this chapter the nurse will:

- Be able to carry out a comprehensive assessment of a patient's pain experience and understand the importance of patient-centeredness within a partnership of care and decision making;

- Be knowledgeable about the commonly used analgesics and understand the multi-modal approach to pain relief; and

- Have a comprehensive knowledge of the biopsychosocial interventions as non-pharmacological approaches to pain relief.

Introduction

So far we have:

- Discussed what the word 'pain' means and have investigated an array of pain assessment tools;

- Looked at what the research has said on pain after day surgery and have highlighted the misconceptions of pain experience which many day surgery patients have; and

- Discussed the accountability issue and have concluded that the nurse is, to a large extent, responsible for assessing and managing patients' pain as he/she spends the longest period of time with them and will ultimately be responsible for their discharge home.

Having agreed that nurses do not always assess and manage post-operative pain as effectively as they might because of barriers that they or the patient bring to the encounter, we are now left wondering how the situation can be made better. Well, this is possible.

If we look first at the gold standard principles of pain assessment and management as set out by the International Association for the Study of Pain (IASP, 1994), we see many similarities between these principles and what has been discussed in the previous chapters. In Chapter 2, we agreed that:

- Pain is viewed as a multidimensional experience made up of sensory, emotional, cognitive, behavioural and cultural components, all of which can influence pain perception and the way we respond to it;

- The assessment of pain should be considered as an important part of its management and be implemented appropriately and regularly;

- The assessment and management of pain are very much rooted in nursing care and remain important components of the nurse's role. However, this process must involve the patients as partners in their care and should be ongoing; and

- Finally, pain assessment and its management should always be clearly documented. It is important to remember that the assessment process serves as a guide to intervention and not solely as an end in itself.

Assessing post-operative pain after day surgery— the way forward

As soon as the patient arrives back on the ward from the recovery unit, the nurse begins to assess the patient's fitness for discharge home within a few hours. We already know, from earlier discussions in Chapter 1, that severe levels of pain can be experienced and this poses a threat to what would normally be an uneventful discharge had the patient's pain been more effectively controlled. Taking on board these principles, a thorough assessment is therefore central to the successful management of this distressing symptom. Its success is dependent on acknowledging that:

- The patient's pain experience is unique;

- The patient is a partner in the assessment process;

- There must be effective communication; and

- A multidimensional approach to pain assessment is essential.

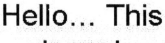

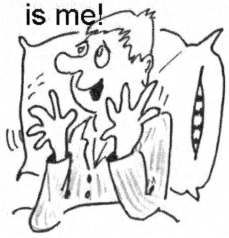

Cartoon 5.2: A unique experience of pain

In the assessment of pain, it is important that, based on the patient's uniqueness of pain experience, an intervention appropriate for each patient and for each episode of pain is identified. The patient should be a partner in the decision-making process. Once more, we are reminded of McCaffery and Beebe's (1989) famous phrase that patients are the experts on their own pain and should therefore be given the opportunity to express the intensity of their pain, as well as what it means to them, in their own words. Kazanowski and Laccetti (2002) describe this communication process between the nurse and the patient as a 'transpersonal relationship' which involves patients sharing knowledge or information about their pain in exchange for high quality nursing care. In this relationship, the nurse takes the lead in providing the structure for the exchange of information and this involves several strategies:

- Privacy is important given that the information exchanged during the assessment is personal and communicated under rather uncomfortable circumstances;

- There should be minimal interruptions as important information may be missed;

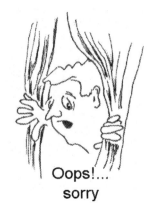

Cartoon 5.3: Privacy

- The assessment interview should be restricted to the pain experience only so that the process will take the least period of time possible and be more productive;

- The interview should also include open ended questions so that patients can freely express their feelings about their pain experience. For example 'How are you feeling now?' and subsequent questions can focus on the type, location, severity and nature of the pain; and

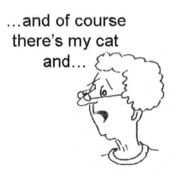

Cartoon 5.4: The time factor

- Finally, it is important for the nurse to have a 'therapeutic presence' (Kazanowiski and Laccetti, 2002) or, as described by Carr and Mann (2000), 'skilled companionship' which involves a caring attitude, receptive body language in which the nurse sits at the same level as the patient, maintaining eye contact and speaking calmly and clearly without using medical jargon, making sure that the language used is understood by the patient.

In Chapter 2, we established that the individual's perception of pain will impact on the emotional, social, familial, occupational and physical functioning of the individual. It is no surprise therefore to find that a multidimensional approach to assessment is required so that the various factors influencing the expression of pain can be identified (Hawthorn and Redmond, 1998). Just as there are nurse and patient barriers that can hinder effective pain management, there are also barriers to the assessment process. These include:

- Anxiety;
- Confusion;
- Physical condition;
- Language and culture; and
- Environment.

Anxiety

There is much research evidence to suggest that the more anxious the patient is, the more pain they are likely to experience (Boore, 1978; Hayward, 1975; Mitchell, 2000) which can affect comprehension, memory and communication skills.

Confusion

This cognitive impairment may be the result of a physiological condition, such as hypotension, hypoxia, hypoglycaemia, or a psychological condition.

Physical condition

The patient may have a hearing or speaking impediment or excessive body weakness.

Language and culture

It is possible that the patient may speak English as a second language and may be compromised in expressing pain verbally. Therefore, there needs to be skilled interpretation of the non-verbal cues which the patient is using. Caution is also needed when family members want to become involved in interpreting, as patient confidentiality should be maintained at all times, and they may not interpret accurately. In addition, culture can also influence the value and meaning of the pain experience and this can range from a stoical attitude in which it is not expressed to an openly vocalised expression of pain.

Environment

In a busy day surgery ward setting, factors such as noise, interruptions and a lack of privacy can have a negative impact on the assessment process.

With the expectation that the nurse is likely to meet some of these barriers, observational and verbal skills are important. Observational skills are essential when patients are cognitively impaired or cannot communicate verbally. We understand this to be subjective data collection about the pain experience. However, assessing pain includes the collection of both subjective and objective data. As discussed in Chapter 2, objective data about the intensity or severity of pain is collected through the use of rating scales and these have been discussed in more detail on pages 23–25, as well as an argument for the use of Visual Analogue Scale (VAS) as an appropriate tool for a day surgery unit. The use of VAS can serve to enhance communication, validate successive interventions and provide more reliable evaluations of these interventions. More importantly, the scale helps us all to 'speak the same language about pain' (Kazanowski and Laccetti, 2002: 23).

Physical assessment

Another method of objective data collection about patients' pain is through physical assessment. A patient's vital signs may show a painful state, for example an increasing pulse and respirations, a decrease in blood pressure and pallor, with the patient becoming increasingly agitated.

A physical assessment would include an evaluation of any redness or swelling. In the day surgery context, this is difficult when the patient has just returned from theatre and the wound has been dressed. However, in some cases, it is necessary to remove the dressings, for example to inspect the wound to check for excessive bleeding. A functional assessment, including sensation and movement of the affected extremity, should also be performed, for example checking the pedal pulse and movement of toes after varicose vein surgery and fingers after carpal tunnel surgery.

Interventions for managing post-operative pain

Once the patient's pain is comprehensively assessed, decisions will need to be made with respect to identifying which strategy can provide optimal relief. Hawthorn and Redmond (1998) contend that, in some ways, the management of acute pain (as is the case here) is less complicated than for chronic pain, since acute pain is transient and is expected to reduce in intensity over a period of time. Within the day surgery context, the problem seems to be one of patients not expecting the severity of pain they go on to experience. This can result in unplanned GP visits (Ghosh and Sallam, 1994; Kong et al, 1997) and require extra physical and emotional support afterwards (Cooper et al, 1995).

The main interventions used to manage pain include:

- Pharmacological (analgesics and opioids);

- Physical (use of touch, massage, heat or cold therapy, transcutaneous stimulation); and

- Behavioural (relaxation, distraction, music therapy, education).

Pharmacological interventions

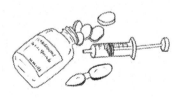

Cartoon 5.5: Pharmacological interventions

We discussed earlier the fact that, although analgesics are prescribed by the doctor, it is the nurse who has to decide on its administration. The nurse's responsibility is based on the five 'R's': the right drug, right dose, right time, right route and right clients. Nurses are responsible for knowing about analgesia in terms of the different doses, effectiveness and side effects and how medications can be combined as a multi-modal approach in providing balanced analgesia. However, our responsibility does not rest there. We also need to be able to educate our patients on the importance of taking analgesia, as some patients do not like to take pain relief, or their side effects.

Analgesics/non-opioids:

Paracetamol/acetaminophen

This is an effective analgesic for mild pain or can be used, for example, with codeine to produce mild to moderate pain relief. It works by inhibiting the body's synthesis of prostaglandin in the CNS (see *Cartoon 2.3*). One of its advantages is that, unlike non-steroidal anti-inflammatory medication (NSAID), it does not produce gastro-intestinal disturbances or affect platelet function. One of the main disadvantages is that it has a limited 'ceiling' and, once this occurs, becomes ineffective. It is also very toxic if more than the recommended dose of eight tablets in 24 hours is taken.

Opioids

These analgesic agents can be used for mild to severe pain and work by binding with opioid receptors in the central and peripheral nervous systems. The main opioids you are more than likely to come across are:

○ Fentanyl, which has a quick onset but is short acting and lasts for about one to two hours;

○ Alfentanil, which has a very rapid onset of about two minutes but will only last for ten minutes;

○ Papaveretum (Omnopom®), which is a much longer acting opioid; and

○ Pethidine, which is commonly used although it has only one tenth of the potency of morphine and lasts between one to three hours.

However, recent research by Lanigan (2001) has argued against the use of pethidine for post-operative pain because of its limitations compared with morphine and its short duration of action. Finally, morphine sulphate is seen as the gold standard for pain relief. These opioids have a twenty minute onset and are effective for between three to four hours. In addition, diamorphine is slightly more potent than morphine and has a faster onset with a shorter duration. The fact that it is soluble in water allows it to be used effectively as an epidural, spinal and intranasal analgesic in the case of ENT surgery. The main advantage of these opioids is that they are highly effective following surgery or trauma during which severe pain is experienced. A second advantage is that they can be used with medication such as paracetamol, aspirin or other NSAIDs to enhance the activity of the opioid.

The main disadvantages of using opioids are the side effects, which include respiratory depression, sedation, nausea and vomiting, confusion, pruritus and constipation. There is no doubt that respiratory depression is the most life-threatening side effect and occurs during parenteral adminis-tration. This side effect is unlikely to occur within the day sur-gery context given that any amount of opioid administered would be closely monitored. Furthermore, there is an expec-tation that the patient will return home on the same day. It is also worth mentioning that pain is a stimulus to respiration so the side effects can only occur once pain is under control (Hawthorn and Redmond, 1998). Should an opioid overdose occur, naloxone or Narcan® should always be at hand to reverse these effects and is administered as a 0.2 micro-gram dose intra-muscularly. It is also useful for pruritus which can develop if the administration of antihistamine proves to be ineffective.

Nausea and vomiting are common side effects following administration of an opioid and are likely to occur in about 30 per cent of patients (O'Brien, 1993: cited by Hawthorn and Redmond, 1998). These symptoms are caused by stimulation of the chemoreceptor trigger zone affecting gastric motility and emptying. The administration of an anti-emetic such as ondansetron has an onset of one hour and can last up to twelve hours. Metoclopramide is also commonly used with an onset of one hour with six to eight hours duration. Other anti-emet-ics with varying hours of duration include prochlorperazine (three to six hours), promethazine (eight to sixteen hours) and chlorpromazine (eight to twelve hours).

The weaker opioids will include codeine phosphate, dihydrocodeine and dextropropoxyphene. Codeine is derived from the opium plant although less potent than morphine and lasts between two to four hours. It is generally administered as a 30 or 60mg dose and often combined with paracetamol. For example, co-codamol is a combination of codeine and paracetamol; co-proxamol is a combination of paracetamol and dextropropoxyphene. Although a weak opioid, when used in this combination, it is effective for moderate pain. Its main disadvantage is that codeine can cause constipation, light-headedness, nausea and vomiting. Dihydrocodine, although a derivative of codeine, is more potent and can be used for mild to moderate pain. Finally, dextropropoxyphene is also a weak opioid but can provide mild to moderate pain relief and is used in combination with paracetamol. Although this drug has a similar side effect to codeine, problems of constipation are less apparent. However, there has been a lot of recent media coverage with regard to this analgesic agent as it is very easy to overdose on it. A report in the Daily Telegraph (Doyle, 2005) stated that about 300–400 people in England and Wales die annually after exceeding the recommended dose. This report has also indicated that one in five of these deaths is due to accidental overdose. Taking two doses more than the recommended eight tablets daily is sufficient to cause death. As a result, the Medicines and Healthcare Regulatory Agency has now recommended that it is withdrawn.

Non-steroidal anti-inflammatory agents (NSAID)

These agents include aspirin, ibuprofen, naproxen, diclofenac and ketorolac and directly act on the wound site by reducing swelling, muscle tenderness or joint stiffness. This is achieved by affecting the body's synthesis of prostaglandin in a very similar way to that of paracetamol. However, in this case, it is the site of tissue damage which is directly affected and this action lasts for three to four hours. The main disadvantage of using this preparation is that there is a ceiling effect, thus taking more will be pointless and may cause dangerous side effects, including:

- Gastro-intestinal toxicity;
- Renal and hepatic problems; and
- Bleeding which generally occurs after long-term use but can occur at any time.

Gastro-intestinal disturbances such as heartburn, gastritis, ulcer formation, perforation and bleeding are very common, thus it is important that these medications are not taken on an empty stomach. Renal and hepatic problems are generally the result of long-term use, particularly in the elderly.

Aspirin

This is possibly one of the world's safest and least expensive analgesic agents and has been used effectively for over 100 years. It is a member of the family of chemicals called salicylates and originates from the willow bark. It is also an antipyretic agent and is effectively used for mild to moderate pain, fever, redness and swelling and to prevent blood from clotting. It works effectively on headaches, infections and arthritis as well as gout. It is also used to prevent a second heart attack or stroke. However, its main disadvantage is that it causes gastro-intestinal problems and can inhibit platelet aggregation. It is therefore not recommended for patients on anti-coagulation therapy. Caution is also needed for patients as there is a 5–10 per cent risk that aspirin can cause a severe asthmatic attack.

World Health Organization analgesic ladder (1990)

Now that the main analgesic agents have been introduced, it is worth mentioning the World Health Organization (1990) three-step analgesic ladder which is widely used to treat pain. Initially, each patient will start at the bottom of the ladder and progress upwards depending on their condition and at which stage the pain is controlled. Although predominantly used for patients with cancer, the ladder provides an effective way of increasing pain control for each of the three steps based on the use of non-opioids, weak opioids and strong opioids (Hawthorn and Redmond, 1998). Firstly, at the bottom of the ladder, non-opioid analgesics are administered and are generally effective in controlling mild pain and which can be supplemented with adjuvants such as NSAIDs as explained earlier. If step one proves to be ineffective, a weak opioid is the next analgesic choice. This can be given as well as the non-opioid to maximise pain control and supplemented with adjuvants. If pain continues to persist and is increasing, the use of a strong opioid is needed. Similarly, these analgesics can also be given

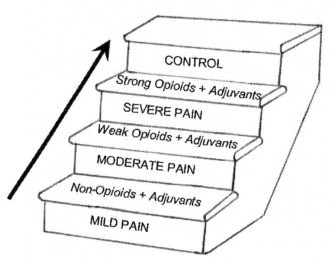

Cartoon 5.6: The WHO analgesic ladder

with non-opioids.

A multi-modal approach

The cartoon at the beginning of this chapter mentioned a multi-modal approach to pain treatment. This means that a combination of different drugs can be administered via different routes as opposed to a single drug, to maximise the analgesic power. A common combination which is used is that of an NSAID and an opioid. For example, the use of co-codamol (30mg/500mg paracetamol) and 50mg diclofenac can be effective for moderate to severe pain. Recent research by Lau *et al* (2002) has contended that the use of pre-emptive analgesia by the administration of diclofenac suppository can spare

OPIOID + NSAID =
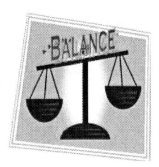

Cartoon 5.7

the use of opioids and their side effects. They found that the use of a 50mg suppository proved to be as equally effective as 30mg IV ketorolac after day case inguinal hernia repair. This has important cost implications as it is argued that diclofenac is about a sixth of the cost of ketorolac.

In addition to the post-operative oral opioid and non-opioid analgesics, balanced analgesia would also commonly involve intra-operative administration of short acting opioids, for example fentanyl and wound infiltration with local anaesthetic, thus ensuring that the patient is comfortable. It is important, however, that the patient is given the appropriate analgesia and clear instructions so that an acceptable level of pain experience can be maintained once the wound infiltration wears off.

The following table is an example of a typical day surgery protocol of analgesics prescribed and administered to patients on their discharge. As you will see, the potency of analgesia varies accordingly to the predicted severity of the pain experience for different day surgical procedures and is in line with the WHO analgesic ladder protocol of using combinations of non-opioids, opioids and adjuvants.

Table 5.1: A typical protocol of analgesics administered in a day surgery unit

Category 1	Analgesia	Paracetamol 500mg x 2 qds (n=50 tablets)
	Procedure	Nasal surgery Antral lavage Myringotomies +/- Grommits Minor peripheral surgery Cystoscopy Cataract extraction
Category 2	Analgesia	Co-codamol 30mg codeine/500mg paracetamol x 1-2 capsules qds (n=30 tablets)
	Procedure	Breast lump Varicose veins Adult circumcision Squint surgery STOP Dilatation and curretage Hysteroscopy TCER
Category 3	Analgesia	Co-codamol 30mg codeine/500mg paracetamol x 1-2 capsules qds (n=30 tablets) + diclofenac 50mg tds (n=28)
	Procedure	Laparoscopy Anal surgery Hernia repair Testicular surgery
Category 4	Analgesia	Tramadol 50mg x 2 capsules qds (n=50 tablets) + paracetamol 500mg qds (n=50) + diclofenac 50mg tds (n=28)
	Procedure	Laparoscopic cholecystectomy TVT (Tension free vaginal tape) Vaginal hysterectomy Orthopaedic procedures

Non-pharmacological interventions

Now that the main pharmacological interventions have been explored, it is important that credence is given to the non-pharmacological interventions which are physical and behavioural approaches. When these are used in combination with pharmacological interventions, they can effectively and holistically address the physical, emotional and cognitive components of the pain experience.

Physical interventions

It is surprising how effective physical interventions can be in providing pain relief. These include:

- Touch and change in position;
- Massage;
- Hot or cold therapy; and
- Transcutaneous electrical nerve stimulation (TENS).

Touch and change in position

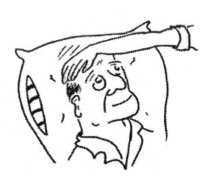

Cartoon 5.8: A sense of touch

The use of touch is in itself therapeutic as it gives the patient a sense of reassurance and will help the patient to relax thereby reducing tension. Helping the patient to change position can also be beneficial to enable improved circulation. Kazanowski and Laccetti (2002) rightly maintain that a patient in pain is generally reluctant to move for fear that their pain will increase. Teaching the patient how to position comfortably in addition to pharmacological interventions ensures that the patient will have an acceptable level of pain and can recover quickly.

Massage

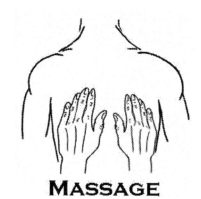

Cartoon 5.9: Massage

This form of touch works by stimulating the skin gently or more vigorously in which A-beta fibres become activated by closing the gate (see *Cartoon 2.5*). This stops the pain impulses from A-delta and C-fibres from reaching the central nervous system (Carr and Mann, 2000) and promotes muscle relaxation. Research by Hulme *et al* (1999) showed that the use of foot massage proved to be beneficial for women undergoing laparoscopic sterilisation.

The use of complementary medicine including Aromatherapy, Reiki and Acupuncture have greatly increased over the last twenty years. It is now estimated that between twenty and 75 per cent of all adults have used at least one type of complementary medicine during the last year (Ernst, 2004). However, with so little research on the role of this approach in pain control, few preliminary conclusions can be drawn, so the jury is out on this one! It is possible that Aromatherapy can be effective as a relaxation response. It is also possible that Acupuncture might work through complicated neuro-physiological pathways. Yet despite this uncertainty, our expenditure on complementary medicine in the UK alone is £1.6 billion (Ernst, 2004).

Hot or cold therapy

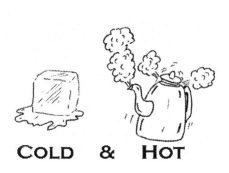

COLD & HOT

Cartoon 5.10: Hot and cold therapy

Heat therapy works by vasodilatation to the specific area where heat is applied; circulation is maximised promoting the removal of toxins and extracellular fluid from the area of tissue injury, thus effectively reducing swelling.

Cold therapy works by numbing the area during which the sensation of cold is conveyed as a message to the central nervous system by 'short circuiting' the gate control mechanism for pain (Kazanowski and Laccetti, 2002). Due to a decrease in body temperature, vasoconstriction occurs causing a reduction in local circulation restricting the amount of extracellular fluid leaking into the area, thus reducing swelling.

For both types of therapy the rule of thumb is for twenty minutes application and then twenty minutes off. Care should be taken not to directly expose skin to ice to prevent tissue damage.

Transcutaneous electrical nerve stimulation (TENS)

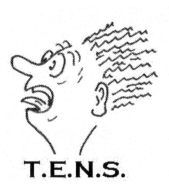

Cartoon 5.11: Transcutaneous electrical nerve stimulation

This device consists of a non-invasive method in which a mild electrical current through a series of pulses is passed across the skin via four electrodes to the superficial nerves near the location of the pain. The electrical stimulations are thought to excite the A-beta fibres which are responsible for closing the gate control mechanism of pain causation and stimulating the production of endorphins (Carr and Mann, 2000).

Behavioural interventions

These interventions include the use of relaxation, distraction, music therapy and patient education and can be effective in reducing pain experience. However, given the transience of the day surgery stay, it is likely that these strategies would be more effective once the patient is back in the comfort of his/her own home.

Relaxation

This intervention combines both physical and behaviour methods and involves the use of controlling one's breathing with exercises and is seen to be effective in reducing tension through the release of endorphins (Kazanowski and Laccetti, 2002).

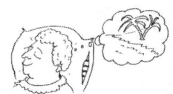

Cartoon 5.12: Relaxation

Distraction

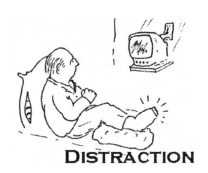

Cartoon 5.13: Distraction

This is a method by which the mind focuses on pleasant stimuli as opposed to pain or negative thoughts (McCaffery and Beebe, 1994: cited by Carr and Mann, 2000). These strategies can include being with other people, reading, watching television or listening to music. Indeed, music therapy is another method and there is evidence that music can promote relaxation and reduce pain. For example, research in the US by Good *et al* (2001) conducted secondary analysis of an experiment that was carried out between 1995 and 1997 of abdominal surgical patients in five hospitals. In this study, groups of patients were either exposed to relaxation, music, a combination of both or a control. Post-operative pain experience on days one and two were measured by VAS and it was concluded that nurses can safely employ any of these interventions for pain on both post-operative days.

Patient and carer education

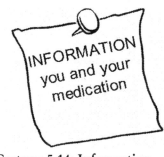

Cartoon 5.14: Information

None of these behavioural therapies can be effective without patient and carer education. This is an important behavioural intervention in its own right. We already know that if patients are treated as a partner in their care and informed about their management, they are likely to cope better. For example, if patients were given realistic expectations about the likely level of pain they will experience after surgery, the likelihood is that their recovery at home and return to work will be quicker than those who had not expected the severity of pain they experienced. In the day surgery context, this positive approach starts at patients' pre-operative assessment in which they should be informed about the surgical technique, the amount of pain likely to be experienced and why this is so, the type of analgesia they will be given and how they should take their analgesia at home after discharge. This educative process can only be effective if it is performed by an experienced, pre-operative assessment nurse who is able to assess the patient's informational needs on an individual basis and can meet them appropriately and efficiently using simple language.

Depending on personality types, some people will require a lot of information, whereas others will prefer not to receive very much information, even if it is their first operation (Mitchell, 2000). Sometimes a quick guided tour of the unit can do much to allay anxiety about the impending operation day. It is also the case that many patients will not remember very much about their pre-operative assessment as they may have been anxious, so it is important that the patient is provided with written information to take home and digest at their leisure.

The families of patients should not be forgotten when it comes to information giving as they will be the main carers, in the majority of cases, and will be providing physical, psychological and social support. Thus, they need to be informed, particularly when administering analgesia after discharge of the patient. They also need to be informed of the likely side effects and how to deal with them. In doing so, myths and misconceptions held by family members about the taking of analgesia can be effectively dealt with, thus ensuring a positive recovery experience.

The nurse's presence

Finally, another behavioural interaction which needs to be mentioned is that of the nurse's presence in being able to stay with the patient in pain which can help the patient to cope better with the experience. Carr and Mann (2000) frequently describe this as being 'skilled companionship'. The benefits of holding the patient's hand and 'being there' should not be underestimated.

Assessment and management of pain after day surgery: the main recommendations

On the basis of what we have discussed in this chapter, it is possible to establish a set of recommendations at every stage of the day surgery process which may help in ensuring that the patient's experience of pain after day surgery is kept to a comfortable level and does not impede the recovery process.

Information giving at the pre-operative assessment

- Information needs should be assessed on an individual basis and provided accordingly;

- Patients need to be aware that different operation types will have different trajectories of pain and require different management strategies;

- Patients need to be more informed of the short-term post-operative pain they are likely to experience immediately after surgery and after their discharge home, so that they have realistic expectations;

- Patients should plan for more support and more time off work;

- The provision of a programme of anxiety management; and

- The provision of written information to support and reiterate what is discussed at the pre-operative assessment.

Post-operative pain assessment

- The assessment of pain should be performed on an individual basis and involve the patient;
- The use of observational as well as verbal skills is important; and
- The introduction of a formalised protocol of pain assessment in each unit.

Post-operative pain management

- Pain intensity and relief must be assessed and re-assessed at regular intervals rather than on a pro rata need basis;
- The use of a multi-modal approach combining short-acting opioids and NSAIDS; and
- The use of non-pharmacological interventions when considered appropriate.

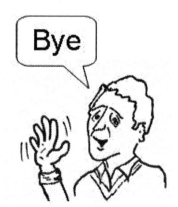

Cartoon 5.15: The discharge

The discharge

- An assessment of pain before discharge;
- Patients need to be informed that it is easier to prevent pain than to chase and reduce it once it has been established;
- Patients should be 'debriefed' before their discharge about what has happened and be provided with specific discharge instructions regarding their pain and the appropriate management of it;

- Appropriate analgesia to take home according to the level of anticipated pain experience; and

- Patient and carer education about taking analgesia and possible side effects.

Post discharge

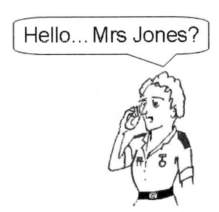

Cartoon 5.16: The post-discharge telephone call

- A nurse-led telephone service for all patients on the day after surgery and a help line to provide reassurance and re-emphasise advice about pain relief;

- A day surgery nurse visiting service for selected patient groups at home to maintain continuity of care and provide advice on pain relief, and to check wound sites; and

- The introduction of a day surgery patient forum in which patients are invited to attend and provide feedback on their day surgical experiences.

Summary

In this chapter we have looked at the importance of pain assessment and the potential barriers that can hinder this process. A comprehensive assessment of the patient's pain experience using pharmacological as well as non-pharmacological interventions has been presented and has addressed the biopyschosocial needs of the patient. Main recommendations, at every stage of the day surgery process from pre-operative to post-discharge, have also been made.

Post-operative pain continues to exist and it is clear from the literature discussed in Chapter 3 that important levels of pain are experienced by day surgery patients for what we would describe as the most common types of day surgical procedures, i.e. laparoscopic sterilisation, hernia and varicose vein surgery. But what are the implications for day surgery as the boundaries of surgical expertise and anaesthetic advancements continue to evolve? The next chapter looks to the future of day surgery and asks the question 'What does the future hold?'

Further reading

Cahill H, Jackson I (1997) *Day Surgery—Principles and Nursing Practice*. Bailliere Tindall, London

Kazanowski MK, Laccetti MS (2002) *Nursing Concepts—Pain*. Slack Incorporated, New Jersey

Sutherland E (1996) *Day Surgery—A Handbook for Nurses*. Bailliere Tindall, London

6

What does the future hold?

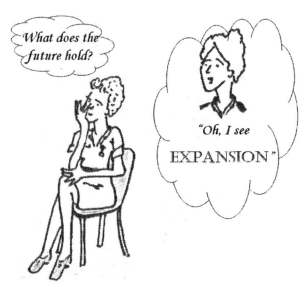

Cartoon 6.1: What does the future hold?

Learning outcomes

At the end of this chapter the nurse will:

- Have a comprehensive knowledge of new surgical and anaesthetic techniques which are currently available or about to be introduced to day surgery;

- Understand the political and economic imperatives behind the expansion of day surgery; and

- Understand the need to address severe levels of pain experience for the more common day surgical procedures before more complex techniques are introduced.

Introduction

Any future expansion of day surgery is dependent on two main factors. Firstly, many technological developments (Cartoon 6.2) have taken place within the fields of anaesthesia and analgesia which are to be (if not already) implemented in day surgery; and secondly, there are the political imperatives (Cartoon 6.3) behind this expansion. Over the last few years, there has been an increasing political interest in day surgery as a means of reducing elective surgical waiting lists.

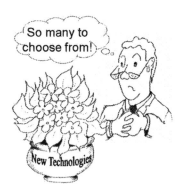

Cartoon 6.2: Technological developments

In 2002, nearly 3.2 million day case operations were carried out which is almost 50 per cent of all operations undertaken in the NHS and this figure is set to rise. In the US, it is estimated that 95 per cent of elective intra-abdominal surgery is performed endoscopically. With these factors in mind, this chapter will explore the implications of these developments on the future of day surgery.

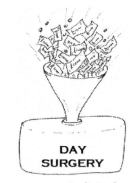

Cartoon 6.3: Political imperatives

New developments

The rapid development of minimally invasive surgery, including the use of laparoscopic techniques, will inevitably mean that there are going to be major changes ahead within day surgery (Wickham, 1994). Technology has brought about the application of robotics (Cartoon 6.4) which now allows surgeons to perform surgical procedures by remote control. Given that these minimally invasive procedures will result in reduced trauma to the patient, this will ultimately reduce the length of hospitalisation so the patient can look forward to going home earlier. This will also have a positive impact on the rate of hospital acquired infections. The consequence of this development will mean that the traditional surgical ward arrangement will soon become redundant. As many patients will not require or indeed want to stay in hospital, it is likely that day surgery will become the surgery of the future and will expand to meet these demands.

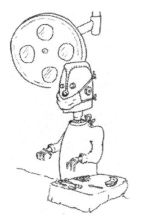

Cartoon 6.4: The application of robotics

In 1994, Wickham predicted that the following would be suitable for day surgical procedures:

- Endoscopic cholecystectomy;

- Endoscopically assisted hysterectomy;

- Endoscopic endometrial ablation;

- Appendicectomy;

- Hernia repair;

- Pulmonary resection;

- Transuretheral prostatic resection;

- Extracorporeal shockwave lithotripsy; and

- Percutaneous endoscopic nephrolithotomy.

Five years later, Wickham's prediction was confirmed when the British Association of Day Surgery (BADS) (1999) proposed a 'trolley' (Cartoon 6.5) of new procedures suitable for day surgery in which many of the procedures indicated by Wickham were considered viable as day cases.

- Laparoscopic cholecystectomy (interval appendicectomy);
- Laparoscopic herniorrhaphy;
- Thoracoscopic sympathectomy;
- Submandibular gland excision;
- Partial thyroidectomy;
- Superficial parotidectomy;
- Breast cancer wide excision with axillary clearance;
- Haemorrhoidectomy;
- Urethrotomy;
- Bladder neck incision;

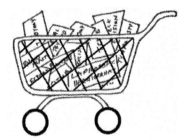

Cartoon 6.5: A trolley of procedures

- Laser prostatectomy;
- Trans cervical resection endometrium (TCRE);
- Eyelid surgery including tarsoplasty, blepharoplasty;
- Hallux valgus ('bunion') operations;
- Arthroscopic menisectomy;
- Arthroscopic shoulder surgery (subacromial decompression);
- Subcutaneous mastectomy;
- Rhinoplasty;
- Dentoalveolar surgery; and
- Tympanoplasty.

With the development of under 24 hour surgery, more complex surgery, including pulmonary lobectomy, prostatectomy and minor craniectomy procedures, will soon be performed as day surgery (Rawal, 2001). Major advances in anaesthetic techniques, including the use of short-acting anaesthetic agents and an increase in the use of regional as opposed to general anaesthesia, will support these developments.

Regional anaesthesia

This type of anaesthesia can greatly reduce or avoid the hazards of having a general anaesthetic, i.e. sore throat, airway trauma and muscle pain. It can provide prolonged post-operative analgesia without sedation and can facilitate earlier discharge. Local or regional anaesthesia can be used independently, in combination with sedation techniques or as part of a balanced analgesia approach with general anaesthesia. Local anaesthetic techniques are simple. They have a high success rate and fewer complications as they limit the systemic side effects of analgesia, such as post-operative nausea and vomiting. Additional benefits include the reduced need for oral opioids, decreased incidence of breakthrough pain and a quicker return to normal activities for the patient.

An example of an innovative method of drug delivery is that of local anaesthetic wound, joint and plexus infusions. This involves the use of an elastomeric balloon pump (Cartoon 6.6) which allows the continuous infusion, or for the patient to self-administer local anaesthetic analgesia whilst at home. The technique involves placing a special catheter subcutaneously into the surgical wound. The catheter is designed with multiple openings so that the drug is able to seep into the wound site along its incision. The balloon pump is filled with a volume of local anaesthetic which allows an infusion for 24–48 hours or enough for self-administration for about ten doses. Post-operatively, when experiencing pain, the patient is able

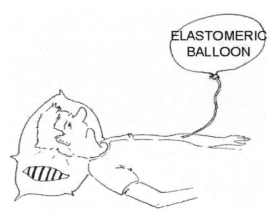

Cartoon 6.6: A continuous infusion balloon pump

to administer a bolus of local anaesthetic by pressing a button which delivers a pre-set volume of the infusion. To stop the infusion, the clamp is closed after the prescribed time (about six minutes). When the analgesia is no longer required, the patient simply removes the tape holding the catheter in place, pulls it out and discards the pump. The main analgesics which are used are bupivacaine or ropivacaine. Examples of continous local analgesia using the infusion pump approach are shown in the next table.

Table 6.1: Examples of local anaesthetic infusions

Author	Procedure	Analgesic agent
Fredman *et al* (2000)	Caesarean delivery	Ropivacaine
Cheong *et al* (2001)	Laparotomy	Bupivacaine
Zohar *et al* (2001)	Total abdominal hysterectomy and bilateral salpingo-oophorectomy	Bupivacaine
Vintar *et al* (2002)	Inguinal hernia repair	Bupivacaine and ropivacaine
Gottschalk *et al* (2003)	Shoulder surgery	Ropivacaine
Gupta *et al* (2004)	Abdominal hysterectomy	Levo-bupivacaine

Over the past few years, there has been an increase in the use of non-invasive approaches in pain management. These have included the use of opioids via different methods of administration. For example, opioids can be introduced through the oral mucosa with the use of oral transmucosal fentanyl. Transnasal sufentanil, fentanyl and meperidine can also be administered. For the skin, transdermal fentanyl and sufentanil can be used and allowed to permeate with the use of an electric current which is called ionotophoresis.

Integrated care pathways

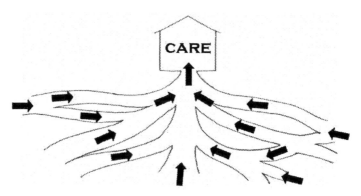

Cartoon 6.7: A pathway of integrated care

Integrated care pathways (ICP) that include anaesthetic technique are set to be used more widely in day surgery units. An ICP is a multidisciplinary outline of 'anticipated' care within a time frame so that the patient is able to move progressively through a clinical experience to a final positive outcome (Middleton *et al*, 2001). ICPs are important as they help to reduce unnecessary variations in patient care and outcomes, for example by using standard anaesthetic techniques and standard agreed analgesics. This is essential in removing variability so that procedures such as laparoscopic cholecystectomy, tonsillectomy and major shoulder and knee procedures can be performed successfully (Personal communication, Dr Ian Jackson, Consultant Anaesthetist, 2005).

Political imperatives

Now that some of the clinical developments have been introduced, which are set to increase the level of day surgery performed, it is important to acknowledge the political and financial imperatives behind the expansion of day surgery. On an optimistic note, it appears that the government is now prepared to invest more resources in this area. In 2002, John Hutton, the Health Minister, confirmed investment in three key areas relating to day surgery. Firstly, £39m was invested for ten more fast-track Diagnostic and Treatment Centres increasing the number of patients treated to over 25,000 a year. Secondly, £22m was allocated to fund 100 schemes to improve access by expanding primary care services and thirdly, the development of one-stop primary care centres in rural and urban areas—the GP surgeries of the future.

The government is now realising that day surgery is an important option for making the NHS more efficient and more convenient for patients. One indication of this was the launching of the National Day Surgery Programme in 2003 as an attempt to drive day surgery forward. As part of the team, it is envisaged that Clinical Champions will work at Strategic Health Authorities (SHAs) to help change practice locally and to devise methods of increasing day surgery rates. In doing so, the programme will support SHAs/trusts to increase the efficiency of the NHS by 'facilitating' shifts from inpatient to day surgery, outpatient to primary care and increasing day surgery productivity overall (Penn, 2003).

The introduction of under 24 hour day surgery continues to expand and in some units 80 per cent plus of elective surgery (excluding endoscopy) is being performed which is above the anticipated 75 per cent by 2010 as predicted by the Department of Health (2000). It is envisaged therefore that surgical services will be reconfigured to become more streamlined so that all 'short-stay surgery' will be at one part of the hospital and all critical care, high dependency units and major surgery will be at another location, with the appropriate level of staffing (Personal communication, Dr Ian Jackson, Consultant Anaesthetist, 2005).

The General Practitioner Contract

Another important factor that may well have a positive impact on day surgery is that by 2005, all patients and their GPs will be able to book hospital appointments at a time and place which is convenient for them. Such options will include attending local or other NHS hospitals, NHS or independent sector treatment centres, private or even international hospitals. Furthermore, GPs and referring consultants will be able to book appointments online (Cartoon 6.8). For the budget holders, day surgery is a more economically viable option. For patients, they have a choice in terms of when and where to have their surgery. For most, it is likely that they will choose day surgery as it does not involve a long waiting list, they can have their surgery on a date which is convenient to them and they can return to the comfort of their own bed afterwards.

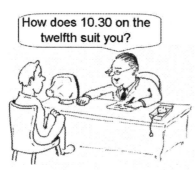

How does 10.30 on the twelfth suit you?

GP/Patient Arrangements

Cartoon 6.8: Booking a day surgery appointment online

So, can I make it better?

Set against this backdrop of technological wizardry and promises of increased funding, and the increased accommodation of patient preference, the question remains whether the day surgery patient experience of post-operative pain can be improved. Yet uncontrolled pain remains the major symptom experienced by patients, particularly after their discharge home, and continues to pose a challenge for all healthcare professionals—particularly as the complexity of day surgical procedures is about to increase. As was shown in Chapter 3, the more recent studies on day surgery pain experience do not show lower levels of pain than the earlier ones.

Although one could be forgiven for being pessimistic at this point, McQuay and Moore (1998) maintain that education is the key for all healthcare professionals involved in the care of day surgery patients, both at pre-registration and post-registration levels. It is our responsibility as healthcare professionals to provide effective pain control and to educate our patients by dispelling myths and misconceptions about pain. As we discussed earlier, this argument is particularly important for day surgery as many patients believe that day surgery is associated with minor surgery and equated with minor symptoms. This is certainly one myth which we need to dispel.

As part of this educative process, working groups of day surgery nurses should be formulated with the aim of collaborating with nurse academics (Cartoon 6.9) to establish more effective pain management interventions. Furthermore, nurses need to work more closely with other clinical services such as pharmacy to improve the quality of pain control.

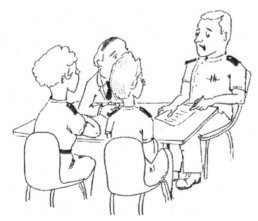

Cartoon 6.9: A working group of day surgery nurses and nurse academics.

Finally, we as healthcare professionals need to keep our knowledge and skills up to date by accessing the evidence as a way of improving our practice; after all, it is part of our code of conduct (NMC, 2002). One way to achieve this would be through the introduction of a pain monitoring programme for nurses and doctors in their daily clinical practice as revision and reinforcement of pain management strategies.

Kalil Gibran (1923) makes the wise observation that:

'Your pain is the breaking of the shell that encloses your understanding.'

(Kalil Gibran, 1923: p61)

This book has enshrined an endeavour to expand that understanding from those who experience pain to those who stand alongside the sufferer. Achieving a position of strength in effective pain management should be the ultimate goal of all day surgery nurses. Only then are we able to say, yes, I **CAN** make it better!

Further reading

Audit Commission (2001) *Day Surgery: Review of National Findings*. Number 4. Audit Commission Publications, London

Cahill J (1999) Basket cases and trollies: day surgery proposals for the millennium. *J One Day Surgery* 9(1): 11–12

Jarrett PEM (1997) Day case surgery: past and future growth. *Surgery* 15(4): 94–96

Glossary

Adjuvant	An additive that enhances the effectiveness of medical treatment.
Axon	Part of the nerve fibre that generally conducts impulses away from the body of the nerve cell.
Bradykinin	A polypeptide which is made up of amino acids and controls the inflammatory response, increases vasodilation and causes contraction of smooth muscle.
CNS	Central Nervous System
Leukotreines	Physiologically active substances involved in the inflammation process and allergic responses.
Myelin sheath	This is the insulating material which surrounds the core of a nerve fibre or axon and is responsible for the transmission of nerve impulses.
NSAID	Non-Steroidal Anti-Inflammatory Drug
Opioid	A synthetic potent drug which is effective in treating moderate to severe pain.
Propagation	The spread of the action potential down an axon that is caused by successive destabilizations of the neuronal membrane.
Prostaglandin E	A hormone-like substance involved in controlling blood pressure, muscle contractions and inflammation.

Substance P	A neurotransmitter which is found in both the central and peripheral nervous systems and involved in the transmission of pain causing rapid contractions of the gastro-intestinal smooth muscle as well as modulating inflammatory and immune responses.
The Numerical Rating Scale	A measurement scale based on numbers like '0', '1', '2', .. to describe the level of patient's pain.
The Verbal Rater/ Descriptor Scale	A measurement scale based on verbal descriptors like 'none', 'mild', 'moderate' and 'severe'.
The Visual Analogue Scale	A continuous measurement scale of 100 mm length with verbal descriptors at each end.

References

Agboola O, Davies J, Davies C (1999) Laparoscopic sterilisation: The immediate and long-term post-operative side effects using bupivacaine infiltration and diclofenac. *J One Day Surg* Winter 98/99: 7–9

American Society of Anesthesiologists (1963) New classification of physical status. *Anesthesiol* 24: 111–12

Audit Commission (2001) *Day Surgery: Review of National Findings*. Number 4. HMSO, London

Audit Commission (1990) *A Short Cut to Better Services: Day Surgery in England and Wales*. Audit Commission, London

Baccaglini U, Giraldi E, Sorrentino P *et al* (1997) Out-patient surgery of the varicose veins of the lower limbs: personal experience. *Ambulatory Surg* 4: 191–92

BADS (1999) *Basket cases and trollies*: http://www.bads.co.uk/trolley.htm. accessed 2005

Bailey IS, Karran SE, Toyn K *et al* (1992) Community Surveillance of complications after hernia surgery. *Br Med J* 304: 469–71

Banta HD (1993) Implications of minimally invasive therapy. *Aus Clin Rev* 13(2): 83–88

Barthelsson C, Lutzen K, Anderberg B *et al* (2003a) Patients' experiences of laparoscopic fundoplication in day surgery. *Ambulatory Surg* 10:101-107

Barthelsson C, Lutzen K, Anderberg B *et al* (2003b) Patients' experiences of laparoscopic cholecystectomy. *J Clin Nurs* 12(2): 253-259

Beauregard L, Pomp A, Choiniere M (1998) Severity and impact of pain after day-surgery. *Can J Anaesthesia* 45(4): 304-311

Boey WK (1995) Challenges in Ambulatory Surgery: discharge criteria. *Ann Acad Med Singapore* **24**(6): 906-9

Boore J (1978) *Prescription for Recovery*. Royal College of Nursing, London

Briggs M, Dean K (1998) A qualitative analysis of the nursing documentation of post-operative pain management. *J Clin Nurs* **7**(2): 155–63

Broks P (2004) The sounds of a chiming clock: Pain perception and the person. In: *Pain, Passion, Compassion and Sensibility*. A Wellcome Trust Exhibition of the Science Museum. 12 Feb-20 June, London, Wellcome Trust

Brunier G, Carson G, Harrison DE (1995) What do nurses know and believe about patients with pain? Results of a hospital survey. *J Pain Symptom Manage* **10**(6): 436–45

Burumdayal A, MacGowan-Palmer JH (2002) A survey of pain at discharge and anaesethetists' prescribing practice following day case laparoscopic sterilisation. *J One Day Surg* **12**(1):11–13

Byrne M, Troy A, Bradley LA *et al* (1982) Cross-validation of the factor structure of the McGill Pain Questionnaire. *Pain* **13**(2): 193–201

Carr D, Goudas L (1999) Acute pain. *Lancet* **353**: 2051–58

Carr ECJ (1997) Overcoming barriers to effective pain control. *Prof Nurse* **12**(6): 412–16

Carr ECJ, Thomas VJ (1997) Anticipating and experiencing post-operative pain: the patients' perspective. *J Clin Nurs* **6**(3): 191–201

Carr EJ, Mann EM (2000) *Pain: Creative Approaches to Effective Management*. MacMillan Press, London

Cheong WK, Seow-Choen F, Eu KW *et al* (2001) Randomised clinical trial of local bupivacaine perfusion versus parenteral morphine infusion for pain relief after laparotomy. *Br J Surg* **88**(3): 357–59

References

Chung F (1995) Recovery pattern and home readiness after ambulatory surgery. *Anesth Analg* **80**: 896–902

Chung F, Ritchie E, Su J (1997) post-operative pain in ambulatory surgery. *Anesth Analg* **85**(4): 808–16

Chung IS, Sim WS, Kim GS *et al* (2001) Nurses' assessment of post-operative pain: can it be an alternative to patients' self reports? *J Korean Med Sci* **16**(6): 784–88

Clarke E, French B, Bilodeau L *et al* (1996) Pain management knowledge, attitudes and clinical practice: the impact of nurses' characteristics and education. *J Pain Symp Manage* **11**(1): 18–29

Cleeland C, Syrjala K (1992) How to assess cancer pain. In: Turk D, Melzack R, eds. *Handbook of Pain Assessment*. Guilford Press, New York

Closs J (1996) Pain and elderly patients: a survey of nurses' knowledge and experiences. *J Adv Nurs* **23**: 237–42

Coll AM (2001) The Effect of Day Surgery on Patients: Three Operative Conditions in Three Different Geographical Locations. Unpublished PhD Thesis, University of Glamorgan

Coll AM, Ameen J, Mead D (2004a) post-operative pain assessment tools in day surgery: a critical review. *J Adv Nurs* **46**(2): 124–33

Coll AM, Ameen J, Moseley L (2004b) A critical review of reported pain after day surgery. *J Adv Nurs* **46**(1): 53–65

Collins SL, Andrew-Moore R, McQuay HJ (1997) The visual analogue pain intensity scale: what is moderate pain in millimetres? *Pain* **72**(1): 95–97

Cooper GM, Malins AF, Jordan, JA (1995) Laparoscopy as a day-case procedure – the patient's view. *Ambulatory Surg* **3**(2): 61–63

Curtis P, Gartman LA, Green DB (1994) Utilisation of ketorolac tromethamine for control of severe odontogenic pain. *J Endodontics* **20**: 457–59

Cushieri A (1999) Technology for minimal access. *Br Med J* **319**: 1304

De Beer DAH, Ravalia A (2001) post-operative pain and nausea following daycase gynacological laparascopy. *J One Day Surg* **Winter 01-02**: 52–53

De Rond M, De Wit R, Van Dam F (1999) Daily pain assessment: value for nurses and patients. *J Adv Nurs* **29**(2): 436–44

DeLoach LJ, Higgins MS, Caplan AB *et al* (1998) The visual analogue scale in the immediate post-operative period: intrasubject variability and correlation with a numeric scale. *Anesth Analg* **86**: 102–106

Department of Health (2002) *Day Surgery: Operatinal Guide*. Waiting booking and choice, London

Department of Health (2000) *The NHS Plan: A Plan for Reform, A Plan for Investment*. HMSO. London

Dewar AL, Craig K, Muir J *et al* (2003) Testing the effectiveness of a nursing intervention in relieving pain following day surgery. *Ambulatory Surg* **10**(2): 81–88

Donovan M, Dillon P, McGuire L (1987) Incidence and characteristics of pain in a sample of medical-surgical inpatients. *Pain* **30**: 69–78

Doyle, C (2005) Danger in the medicine cupboard. *The Daily Telegraph* 1st February, 2005

Emflorgo CA (1999) The assessment and treatment of wound pain. *J Wound Care* **8**(8): 384–85

Ernst E (2004) Complementary medicine for pain in pain therapy. In: *Pain, Passion, Compassion and Sensibility*. A Wellcome Trust Exhibition of the Science Museum. 12 Feb-20 June, London, Wellcome Trust

Firth F (1991) Pain after day surgery. *Nurs Times* **87**(40): 72–75

Fitzgerald M (2004) Dissecting pain: A personal journey through pain research. In: *Pain, Passion, Compassion and Sensibility*. A Wellcome Trust Exhibition of the Science Museum. 12 Feb-20 June, London, Wellcome Trust

Flaherty SA (1996) Pain measurement tools for clinical practice and research. *J Am Ass Nurse Anesth* 64(2): 133–40

Fortier J, Chung F, Su J (1996) Predictive factors of unanticipated admission in Ambulatory Surgery: a prospective study. *Anesthesiol* 85: A27

Fraser RA, Hotz SB, Hurtig JB *et al* (1989) The prevalence and impact of pain after day-care tubal ligation surgery. *Pain* 39(2): 189–201

Fredman B, Shapiro A, Zohar E *et al* (2000) The analgesic efficacy of patient controlled ropivacaine instillation after Caesarean delivery. *Anesth Analg* 91(6): 1436–40

Ghosh S, Sallam S (1994) Patient satisfaction and post-operative demands on hospital and community services after day surgery. *Br J Surg* 81: 1635–38

Gold BS, Kitz DS, Lecky JH *et al* (1989) Unanticipated admission to the hospital following ambulatory surgery. *JAMA* 262(21): 3008–10

Good M (1999) Acute pain. *Ann Rev Nurs Res* 17: 107–32

Good M, Stanton-Hicks M, Grass JA *et al* (2001) Relaxation and music to reduce post-surgical pain. *J Adv Nurs* 33(2): 208–15

Gottschalk A, Burmeister MA, Radtke P *et al* (2003) Continuous wound infiltration with ropivacaine reduces pain analgesic requirement after shoulder surgery. *Anesth Analg* 97(4):1086–91

Graham C, Bond SS, Gerkovich MM *et al* (1980) Use of the McGill Pain Questionnaire in the assessment of cancer pain: replicability and consistency. *Pain* 8(3): 377–87

Gudex C, Dolan P, Kind P *et al* (1996) Health state valuations from the general public using the Visual Analogue Scale. *Qual Life Res* 5: 521–31

Gupta A, Perniola A, Axelsson K *et al* (2004) post-operative pain after abdominal hysterectomy: A double blind comparison between placebo and local anaesthetic infused intraperitoneally. *Anesth Analg* 99: 1173–79

Hamilton J, Edgar L (1992) A survey examining nurses' knowledge of pain control. *J Pain Sympt Man* 7(1): 18–26

Hardman DTA, Patel MI, Fisher CM *et al* (1995) Experience with Varicose Vein Surgery in a day surgical centre. *Ambulatory Surg* 3(1): 7–11

Hawthorn J, Redmond K (1998) *Pain Causes and Management.* Blackwell, Oxford.

Hayward, J (1975) *Information: A Prescription Against Pain.* Royal College of Nursing, London

Heron E, Lozinguez O (1999) Long term sequelae of spontaneous axillary-subclavian venous thrombosis. *Ann Int Med* 131(7): 510–13

Hitchcock M, Ogg TW (1995) Anaesthesia for day-case surgery. *Br J Hosp Med* 54(5): 202–206

Hulme J, Waterman H, Hillier VF (1999) The effect of foot massage on patients' perception of care following laparoscopic sterilisation as day case patients. *J Adv Nurs* 30(2):460–68

Huskisson EC (1982) Measurement of pain. *J Rheumatol* 9: 768–69

IASP (1994) From: *Classification of Chronic Pain*, (2nd Edition), IASP Taskforce on Taxonomy, edited by H Merskey, N Bogduk, IASP Press, Seattle, 209–14

Jackson I, McWhinnie D (2002) What is a day case? *J One Day Surg* 12(1): 5

Jackson IJB, Paton RH, Hawkshaw D (1997) Telephone follow up the day after day surgery. *J One-Day Surg* Spring: 5–7

Jackson IJB, Blackburn A, Tams J *et al* (1993) Expansion of day surgery : a survey of general practitioners views. *J One Day Surg* Spring: 4–7

James FR, Large RG, Bushnell JA *et al* (1991) Epidemiology of pain in New Zealand. *Pain* 44: 279–83

Jensen MP, Smith DG, Ehde DM *et al* (2001) Pain site and the effects of amputation pain: further clarification of the meaning of mild, moderate and severe pain. *Pain* **91**(3): 317–22

Joshi GP (1994) post-operative pain management. *Int Anesthesiol Clin* **32**(3): 113–26

Kalil Gibran, G (1923) *The Prophet*. Alfred A Knopf, New York

Katz J, Melzack R (1999) Measurement of pain. *Surgic Clin N Am* **79**(2): 231–52

Kazanowski MK, Laccetti MS (2002) *Nursing Concepts – Pain*. Slack Incorporated, New Jersey

Keele KD (1948) The pain chart. *Lancet* **2**: 6–8

Kelly AM (2000) Patient satisfaction with pain management does not correlate with initial or discharge VAS pain score, verbal rating at discharge, or change in VAS score in the emergency department. *J Emerg Med* **19**(2): 113–16

Kelly MC (1994) Patients' perception of day case surgery. *Ulster Med J* **63**(1): 27–31

Kelly H, Bain J, Snadden D (1998) Day surgery and primary care: views from practice nurses. *J One Day Surgery* **Spring**: 5–7

Khan MA, Hall C, Smith I (2002) Day case laparoscopic cholecystectomy preliminary experience. *J One Day Surg* **11**(4): 66–68

Kiley P (2004) On medical screaming. In: *Pain, Passion, Compassion and Sensibility*. A Wellcome Trust Exhibition of the Science Museum. 12 Feb-20 June, London, Wellcome Trust

Kleinman A (1988) *The Illness Narratives: Suffering, Healing, and the Human Condition*. Basic Books, New York

Klepac RK, Dowling J, Rokke P *et al* (1981) Interview vs. paper and pencil administration of the McGill Pain Questionnaire. *Pain* **11**(2): 241–46

Kong KL, Child DL, Donovan IA *et al* (1997) Demand on primary healthcare after day surgery. *Ann Roy Coll Surgeons Engl* **79**(4): 291–95

Lanigan C (2001) Hidden pain after day surgery (letter). *J One Day Surg* 10(4): 9

Lau H, Wong C, Lung C *et al* (2002) Prospective randomised trial of pre-emptive analgesics following ambulatory inguinal hernia repair: Intravenous ketorolac versus diclofenac suppository. *Aus N Z J Surg* 72(10): 704–27

Lawlis GF, Achterberg J, Kenner L *et al* (1984) Ethnic and sex differences in response to clinical and induced pain in chronic spinal pain patients. *Spine* 9: 751–54

Leith SE, Hawkshaw D, Jackson JB (1994) A national survey of the importance and drug treatment of pain and emesis following day surgery. *J One Day Surg* 4(2): 24–25

Lewin J, Razis P (1995) Prescribing practice of take home analgesia for day case surgery. *Br J Nurs* 4(18): 1047–51

Lewis C, Bryson J (1998) Does day case surgery generate extra workload for primary and community health service staff? *Ann Roy Coll Surgeons Eng* 80(3): 200–202

Linden I, Bergbom Engberg I (1995) Patients' opinions and experiences of ambulatory surgery—A Self care perspective. *Ambulatory Surg* 3(3): 131–39

Lloyd G, McLauchlan A (1994) Nurses' attitudes towards management of pain. *Nurs Times* 90(43): 40–43

Loeser, JD (2004) Trends in pain therapy. In: *Pain, Passion, Compassion and Sensibility*. A Wellcome Trust Exhibition of the Science Museum. 12 Feb-20 June, London, Wellcome Trust

Mackintosh C (1994) Do nurses provide adequate post-operative pain relief? *Br J Nurs* 3(7): 342–47

Mackintosh C, Bowles S (1998) Audit of post-operative pain following day surgery. *Br J Nurs* 7(11): 641–45

Marks RM, Sachar EJ (1973) Undertreatment of medical inpatients with narcotic analgesics. *Ann Intern Med* 78(2): 173–81

Marley R, Swanson J (2001) Patient care after discharge from the ambulatory surgical centre. *J PeriAnesth Nurs* 16: 399–419

Marquié L, Raufaste E, Lauque D, Mariné C, Ecoiffier M, Sorum P (2003) Pain rating by patients and physicians: Evidence of systematic pain miscalibration. *Pain* 102(3): 289–96

Marshall S, Chung F (1997) Assessment of 'home readiness': discharge criteria and post-discharge complications. *Curr Opin Anaesthesiol* 10(6): 445–50

McCaffery M, Beebe A (1994) *Pain: Clinical Manual for Nursing Practice*. CV Mosby, London

McCaffery M, Beebe A (1989) *Pain: Clinical Manual for Nursing Practice*. C V Mosby, St Louis, MO

McCaffery M, Ferrel B, Page E (1990) Nurses' knowledge of opioid analgesic drugs and psychological dependence. *Cancer Nurs* 13(1): 21–27

McDonald DD (1994) Gender and ethnic stereotyping and narcotic analgesic administration. *Res Nurs Health* 17: 45–49

McGuire D (1988) Measuring Pain. In: Frank-Stromborg M, ed. *Instruments for Clinical Nursing Research*. Appleton and Lange, California

McGuire DB (1984) Assessment of pain in cancer patients using the McGill Pain Questionnaire. *Oncol Nurs Forum* 11(6): 32

McHugh GA, Thoms GMM (2002) The management of pain following day case surgery. *Anaesthesia* 57: 270–74

McMenemin I (1999) Management of pain after day surgery. *J One Day Surg* Winter: 10–11

McQuay H, Moore R (1998) *An Evidence-Based Resource for Pain Relief*. Oxford University Press, Oxford

Melzack R, Casey KL (1968) Sensory, motivational and central control determinants of pain: A new conceptual model. In: Kenshalo D, ed. *The Skin Senses*. Charles C Thomas, Springfield, IL: 423–39

Melzack R, Wall P (1982) *The Challenge of Pain*. Penguin Books, London

Melzack R, Wall PD (1965) Pain mechanisms: a new theory. *Science* 150: 971–79

Middleton S, Barnett J, Reeves D (2001) What is an integrated care pathway? *Hayward Med Comm* 3(3): 1–7

Mitchell M (2004) Pain management in day case surgery. *Nurs Stand* 18(25): 33–38

Mitchell M (2000) Anxiety management: A distinct nursing role in day surgery. *Ambulatory Surg* 8: 119–27

Moore J, Ziebland S, Kennedy S (2002) People sometimes react funny if they're not told enough: Womens' views about the risks of diagnostic laparoscopy. *Health Expectat* 5(4): 302–309

Nash R, Yates P, Edwards H *et al* (1999) Pain and the administration of analgesia: what nurses say. *J Clin Nurs* 8(2): 180–89

NMC (2002) *Code of Professional Conduct.* Nursing and Midwifery Council, London

Oberle K, Allen M, Lynkowski P (1994) Follow-up of same day surgery patients. A study of patient concerns. *AORN J* 59(5): 1016–18

Padfield D (2004) The body in conflict: The visual representation of chronic pain. In: *Pain, Passion, Compassion and Sensibility.* A Wellcome Trust Exhibition of the Science Museum. 12 Feb-20 June, Wellcome Trust, London

Parlow J, Meikle A, van Vlymen J *et al* (1999) Post discharge nausea and vomiting after ambulatory paraoscopy is not reduced by promethazine prophylaxis. *Can J Anaesthesia* 46: 1–24

Penn, S (2003) The national delivery strategy: http:/www.bads.co.uk/modernisation_agency.html (accessed 01-02-05)

Petticrew M, Black NA, Moore L (1995) Day surgery dilatation and curettage: patients' experiences. *Ambulatory Surg* 3(4): 185–88

Price DD, McGrath PA, Rafii A *et al* (1983) The validation of Visual Analogue Scales as Ratio scale measures for chronic and experimental pain. *Pain* **17**(1): 45–56

Prieto EJ, Hopson L, Bradley LA *et al* (1980) The language of low back pain: factor structure of the McGill Pain Questionnaire. *Pain* **8**(1): 11–19

Quigley C, Joel S, Patel N, Baksh A, Slevin M (2002) A phase 1/11 study of nubilised morphine-6-glucuronide in patients with cancer-related breathlessness. *J Pain Symp Man* **23**(1): 7–9

Rawal N (2001) Analgesia for day case surgery. *Br J Anaesthesia* **87**(1): 73–87

Royal College of Surgeons of England/College of Anaesthetists (1990) *Commission on the Provision of Surgical Services: Report of the Working Party on Pain after Surgery*. RCSCA, London

Rudkin GE, Osborne GA, Doyle CE (1993) Assessment and selection of patients for day surgery in a public hospital. *Med J Aus* **158**(5): 308–12

Sanders MN (1995) Varicose vein day surgery follow up. *J One-Day Surg* **Spring**: 11–12

Saxey S (1986) The nurse's response to post-operative pain. *Nursing* **3**(10): 377–81

Schafheutle EI, Cantrill JA, Noyce PR (2001) Why is pain management suboptimal on surgical wards? *J Adv Nurs* **33**(6): 728–37

Scott J, Huskisson EC (1976) Graphic representation of pain. *Pain* **2**(2): 185–95

Seers K (1987) Perceptions of pain. *Nurs Times* **83**(48): 37–39

Seymour RA, Kelly PJ, Hawkesford JE (1996) The efficacy of ketoprofen and paracetamol (acetaminophen) in post-operative pain after third molar surgery. *Br J Clin Pharmacol* **41**(6): 581–85

Sjostrom B, Dahlgren LO, Haljamae H (2000) Strategies used in post-operative pain assessment and their clinical accuracy. *J Clin Nurs* **9**(1): 111–18

Skilton M (2003) post-operative pain management in day surgery. *Nurs Stand* **17**(38): 39–44

Slappendel R, Weber EN, Bugter ML *et al* (1999) The intensity of pre-operative pain is directly correlated in the amount of morphine needed for post-operative analgesia. *Anesth Analg* **88**(1): 46–48

Stubhaug A, Grimstad J, Breivik H (1995) Lack of analgesic effect of 50 and 100mg oral tramadol after orthopaedic surgery: a randomised double-blind, placebo and standard active drug comparison. *Pain* **62**: 111–18

Tanabe P, Buschmann M (2000) Emergency nurses' knowledge of pain management principles. *J Emerg Nurs* **26**(4): 299–305

Thatcher J (1996) Follow-up after day surgery: how well do patients cope? *Nurs Times* **92**(37): 30–32

Thomas H, Hare MJ (1987) Day case laparoscopic sterilisation—time for a rethink? *Br J Obstet Gynaecol* **94**(May): 445–48

Tittle M, McMillan SC (1994) Pain and pain related side effects in an ICU and on a surgical unit: nurses' management. *Am J Crit Care* **3**(1): 25–30

Tong D, Chung F (1999) post-operative pain control in ambulatory surgery. *Surgic Clin N Am* **79**(2): 401–15

Van Duijn NP (1995) Translations and use of the McGill Pain Questionnaire. *MAPI Res Inst* **12**: 7–9: http://www.mapi-research.fr/pdf/newsletter/qol12 (accessed 10/11/04)

Vintar N, Pozlep G, Rawal N *et al* (2002) Incisional self administration of bupivacaine or ropivacaine provide effective analgesia after inguinal hernia repair. *Can J Anesthesia* **49**: 481–86

Watt-Watson J, Chung F, Chan V *et al* (2004) Pain management following discharge after ambulatory same day surgery. *J Nurs Manage* **12**: 153–61

Weissman D, Gordon D, Bidar-Sielaff S (2002) Cultural aspects of pain management. End of Life Physician Education Resource Center: www.eperc.mcw.edu

Westman L, Ultenius I, Ekblom A (1996a) A follow up study of the post-operative period at the hospital in patients scheduled for one-day surgery. *Ambulatory Surg* 4: 5–9

Westman L, Legeby M, Ekblom A (1996b) A 3-day post-operative study related to pain, nausea, vomiting and tiredness in patients scheduled for day surgery. *Ambulatory Surg* 4: 61–66

Wetchler BV (1997) A quarter century of accepting the challenges while avoiding the pitfalls of ambulatory surgery. *Ambulatory Surg* 5(3): 101–104

White PF (1995) Management of post-operative pain and emesis. *Can J Anaesthesia* 42(11): 1053–55

Wickham JEA (1994) Minimally invasive surgery: Future developments. *Br Med J* 308: 193–95

Wigens L (1997) The conflict between new nursing and scientific management as perceived by surgical nurses. *J Adv Nurs* 25(6): 1116–22

Wilkinson D, Bristow A, Higgins D (1992) Morbidity following day surgery. *J One-Day Surg* 2(1): 5–6

Willis CE, Watson JD, Harper CV *et al* (1997) Does day surgery embarrass the primary health care team? An audit of complications and consultations. *Ambulatory Surg* 5(2): 71–75

Wong DL, Hockenberry M, Wilson D *et al* (2001) *Wong's Essentials of Pediatric Nursing*, 6th edn. Mosby Inc, St Louis

Wood JN, Beggs S, Drew LJ (2004) Sensing damage in pain therapy. In: *Pain, Passion, Compassion and Sensibility*. A Wellcome Trust Exhibition of the Science Museum. 12 Feb-20 June, Wellcome Trust, London

World Health Organization (1990) *Cancer Pain Relief and Palliative Care*. Report of a WHO expert committee [World Health Organization Technical Report Series, 804] World Health Organization, Geneva, Switzerland: 1–75

Yates P, Dewar A, Fentiman B (1995). Pain: the view of elderly people living in long-term residential settings. *J Adv Nurs* **21**: 667–74

Zalon ML(1993). Nurses' assessment of post-operative patients' pain. *Pain* **54**: 329–33

Zohar E, Fredman B, Phillipov A *et al* (2001) The analgesic efficacy of patient controlled bupivacaine wound instillation after total abdominal hysterectomy with bilateral salpingo-oophorectomy. *Anesth Analg* **93**(2): 482–87

List of Contacts

Ambulatory Surgery: www.intl.elsevierhealth.com/journals/amsu

Association of Anaesthetists of Great Britain and Ireland, 21 Portland Place, London WC1B 1PY: www.aagbi.org

British Association of Day Surgery, 35–43 Lincoln's Inn Fields, London, WC2A 3PE: www.bads.co.uk/

Day Surgery Nursing Forum, Royal College of Nursing, RCN Institute, 20 Cavendish Square, London, W1G 0RN

Federated Ambulatory Surgery Association: www.fasa.org/

International Association for Ambulatory Surgery (IAAS): www.iaas-med.org/

Journal of One Day Surgery: www.bads.co.uk/journal.htm/

Royal College of Anaesthetists, 48–49 Russell Square, London WC1B 4JY: www.rcoa.ac.uk

The European Society of Regional Anaesthesia and Pain Therapy: www/esraeurope.org

Index

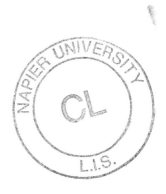

Printed in the United Kingdom
by Lightning Source UK Ltd.
107502UKS00001B/235-294